A COMPLETE GUIDE TO THE FINAL FRCR 2B

A COMPLETE GUIDE TO THE FINAL FRCR 2B

Edited by

Deepak Subedi
MRCP, FRCR
Consultant Radiologist
NHS Fife, Scotland

Marialena Gregoriades
MRCP, FRCR
Consultant Radiologist
NHS Fife, Scotland

En Hsun Choi
MRCP, FRCR
Consultant Radiologist
Stirling Royal Infirmary, Scotland

and

John T Murchison
DMRD, FRCR, FRCP
Consultant Radiologist
Royal Infirmary of Edinburgh, Scotland

Foreword by
Graham McKillop
MRCP, FRCR
Consultant Radiologist
Edinburgh, Scotland

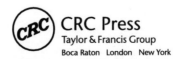

CRC Press
Taylor & Francis Group
Boca Raton   London   New York

CRC Press is an imprint of the
Taylor & Francis Group, an **informa** business

Radcliffe Publishing Ltd
33–41 Dallington Street
London
EC1V 0BB
United Kingdom

www.radcliffepublishing.com

Electronic catalogue and worldwide online ordering facility.

British Library Cataloguing in Publication Data

A catalogue record for this book is available from the British Library.

ISBN-13: 978 184619 447 4

Typeset by Phoenix Photosetting, Chatham, Kent

Contents

Foreword

The FRCR 2B Examination is, for most trainees in Radiology, the final, major medical exam they are required to overcome in their medical career: it is the last major hurdle to clear prior to a consultant post. It is generally taken after 3–4 years of specialised radiological training; at this stage of their career most trainees will have had their fill of exams, will likely have numerous personal commitments outwith work and will be thinking of permanently settling down somewhere.

These factors cause the '2B' to take on an all-encompassing, all-consuming air that means *all* trainees just want it to be over: pass the '2B' and one can start to think about career choices, consultant posts, forgetting studying and becoming a normal creature again outside of work!

Doctors, by-and-large, are a competitive bunch: there is definite peer pressure amongst the trainees working together towards each sitting of the FRCR 2B, absolutely no-one wants to fail. The intensity of preparation this generates includes reading standard textbooks and journals, reviewing cases from film libraries, regular, in-house mock exam sessions, exam-preparation courses and, of course, exam-preparation books.

Writing such a book is no minor undertaking: the task of finding high-quality cases that are unequivocal is daunting; one has to be ruthless in weeding out examples that could cause confusion; and the specimen answers need to be well-nigh perfect to be accepted by the highly motivated exam candidates. Nothing annoys pre-2B trainees more than a case where there is a subtle finding, ignored by those setting the exam, which alters the whole flavour of the answer! The drive exhibited by virtually every pre-exam trainee means their thirst for preparatory work of this type is almost insatiable.

My colleagues have taken on this arduous task to produce *A Complete Guide to the Final FRCR 2B*. The authors constitute three very able, newly-appointed consultants, all of whom have passed their FRCR 2B within the preceding 5 years (while registrars on the Edinburgh-based training scheme), and one very experienced Edinburgh consultant who has just completed his 5-year term as a Royal College of Radiologists' Examiner. This group has produced what is, in my opinion, an excellent exam primer.

The opening section gives a very practical and insightful overview of the actual mechanics of the exam process itself. However, the bulk of the book deals with the crucial task of giving beautiful examples of the type of case commonly encountered in the three components of the exam. The answers proffered are accurate and instructive and will hopefully avoid any irritating equivocation that can be very annoying in the lead-up to the exam.

This book represents a very high-standard addition to the exam preparation book catalogue. Were I to be sitting my FRCR 2B again, I would unequivocally benefit from reading it.

Graham McKillop MRCP, FRCR
Consultant Radiologist
Edinburgh, Scotland
January 2011

Preface

The Part 2B Final Fellowship of the Royal College of Radiologists' examination is taken by UK radiology trainees after three years in a recognised training programme. It is held in London at the College twice a year, normally in the second or third week of April and October. Once a year, usually at the autumn sitting, a Joint Final FRCR/FHKCR Part B Examination for the Fellowship of the Royal College of Radiologists and Hong Kong College of Radiologists is held in Hong Kong. The examination consists of three components, namely *rapid reporting*, a *reporting session* and the *oral examination/viva voce*. The rapid reporting and reporting session are taken together in the same sitting (morning or afternoon), but the viva voce may take place on a different day.

This book is divided into two sections. The first short section consists of advice on how to approach your preparation and the examination itself. The remainder and bulk of the book is divided into the three sections of the examination, with examples of films that you may be shown.

We cannot show you every conceivable condition or film, but hopefully by using this book you will gain sufficient breadth of knowledge to pass well. It is also our intention that, by using this book, candidates who do not have access to teaching or film libraries will have a good chance of passing. We therefore provide you with examples of the common cases shown, as well as giving examples of the more unusual ones.

Deepak Subedi
Marialena Gregoriades
En Hsun Choi
John T Murchison
January 2011

List of image contributors

Dr Deepak Subedi, Consultant Radiologist, NHS Fife, Fife, Scotland

Dr Marialena Gregoriades, Consultant Radiologist, NHS Fife, Fife, Scotland

Dr En Hsun Choi, Consultant Radiologist, Stirling Royal Infirmary, Stirling, Scotland

Dr John T Murchison, Consultant Radiologist, Royal Infirmary of Edinburgh, Edinburgh, Scotland

Dr Stephen Glancy, Consultant Radiologist, Western General Hospital, Edinburgh, Scotland

Dr Fergus J Perks, Consultant Radiologist, Royal Infirmary of Edinburgh, Edinburgh, Scotland

Dr Simon McGurk, Consultant Radiologist, Royal Hospital for Sick Children, Edinburgh, Scotland

Dr Dominic Brown, Consultant Radiologist, Western General Hospital, Edinburgh, Scotland

Dr Awain Yong, Specialist Registrar in Radiology, South East Scotland Training Scheme, Edinburgh, Scotland

Dr Johann DuPlessis, Specialist Registrar in Radiology, South East Scotland Training Scheme, Edinburgh, Scotland

Dr Alan Simms, Specialist Registrar in Radiology, South East Scotland Training Scheme, Edinburgh, Scotland

Dr David Scott, Consultant Radiologist, NHS Fife, Fife, Scotland

Dr Karim Samji, Specialist Registrar in Radiology, South East Scotland Training Scheme, Edinburgh, Scotland

To my parents Keshav and Kalpana Subedi,
my wife Pratima, and my daughter Niharika

DS

Section I

Chapter 1
The examination

Each component is important, but the key is to do well overall. It is not true that you must pass each component individually. Some people have failed the rapid reporting, but do exceedingly well in the other components and have passed overall. A closed marking scheme with marks between 4 and 8 is used for all components (*see* Table 1.1).

Mark	Category
4	Bad fail
5	Fail
6	Pass
7	Good pass
8	Excellent

Table 1.1 Marking scheme

The three components of the examination at the time of publication are described below, but the RCR website should be consulted in order to check whether there have been any changes.

RAPID REPORTING

The rapid reporting section is designed to test your powers of observation and interpretation under time pressure. You have 35 minutes to review 30 images. You will be warned by an invigilator when you are 5 minutes from the end of the exam. These are basically the type of plain X-rays you would see in an Emergency Department reporting session during your normal working day. Of the 30 images, one-third to two-thirds will be normal, with the precise proportion known only to the examiners. The examinations are generally single images, but multiple images (usually two views) may be shown. For each of them you have to record whether the examination is normal or abnormal, and if you think it is abnormal, state what you think the abnormality is. There will only be one abnormality or unifying diagnosis, and anatomical variants or age-related changes are considered normal. A sample answer sheet is shown in Box 1.1. As of the publication of this book, the RCR has moved to an electronic format for rapid reporting and the reporting session. You will be supplied with an Apple Mac Mini and a mouse (but no keyboard). The PACS software is a freeware program OSIRIX, which Mac (but not PC) users can download at home for themselves, in order to practise with it. That said, a short amount of time will be allocated prior to the examination commencing to allow candidates to familiarise themselves with the software. You will be able to window, zoom and pan to review the images. You can also choose to look at the images in sequence or go through them in any order you choose by accessing a list.

A	B	C	D		E		
Case number	Normal	Abnormal	Diagnosis or abnormality (only required if column C is ticked)		Examiner's use only		
01	✓				**1**	**2**	*
02		✓	Fractured right distal radius				
03	✓						
04	✓						
05		✓	Fractured left scapoid				

Box 1.1 Rapid reporting answer sheet (from RCR website)

REPORTING SESSION

Also known as the 'written exam' or 'long cases' by local candidates, this component consists of six cases, each usually containing images of two or more modalities (e.g. X-ray, nuclear medicine and MRI) although on occasions only one modality is provided. As of 2010, a pre-printed answer sheet displaying these headings will be provided (*see* Box 1.2). You do not have to write under every heading. There may not, for example, be a differential diagnosis or any further investigation or management. You will have 55 minutes in which to 'report' the findings. You will be warned by an invigilator when you have 5 minutes until the end of the exam. The college recommendations for the layout of your answer can be found on their website, and will become apparent as you read through this book, but are reproduced in Box 1.3.

Case 1

Age: 72 years	Gender: Male
Clinical problem: Back pain following a fall	
Images in exam case: Plain radiograph (4), CT (2)	

Findings:

Interpretation:

Principal diagnosis:

Differential diagnosis:

Further investigations and management:

Box 1.2 Reporting session answer sheet

> **1 Observations**
> In this section, you should record your observations on the films from all of the imaging studies available to you, including relevant positive and negative findings.
>
> **2 Interpretation**
> Here you should state your interpretation of the observed findings (e.g. describe whether the mass or process you observe is benign, malignant or infective rather than neoplastic, giving your reasons).
>
> **3 Main or principal diagnosis**
> Based on your interpretation you should attempt to reach a single diagnosis. If this is not possible, state here which diagnosis you feel is most likely, and then list the other possibilities, in order of likelihood, in the differential diagnosis section.
>
> **4 Any differential diagnoses**
> For some cases there will be no differential diagnoses, whereas in others you may feel that you wish to include a few. These should be limited in number and brief. In your report you should indicate why you feel that these were less likely than your main or principal diagnosis.
>
> **5 Any relevant further investigations or management**
> In this section you should indicate any further appropriate investigations or clinical management. For example, if you diagnose a patient with a subdural collection, urgent referral is needed if there is evidence of brain compression. Similarly, if you make a diagnosis of an abscess or tumour, you should indicate whether a drainage or biopsy is appropriate.

Box 1.3 Recommended format for reporting session answers (from RCR website)

The RCR states that you can write either in bullet points or in free text.

ORAL EXAMINATION

The viva consists of two separate vivas, in two different rooms. Each viva is conducted by two examiners and lasts 30 minutes. During that time, one examiner will show you their collection of films for 15 minutes while the other examiner remains silent. They will then swap roles for the second 15 minutes, usually after a knock on the door by the invigilator. At the end of the first 30-minute viva, a bell will ring, signalling the end of that viva. You will then move to the next room, where the process will be repeated with another pair of examiners. The oral examination takes a total of one hour.

All of the films are marked individually by both examiners, who agree a consensus final mark once you have left the room.

Films are assessed for observational skills, interpretation of the findings, and management, including safety. There is no minimum number of cases that you have to see in order to pass, but the more films you do see, the greater is the likelihood that you will obtain a good mark. If you see two modalities on one case (e.g. CXR and CT scan), this will generally count as two cases for marking purposes. The examiners will expect a higher level of understanding of the easier films, but will be more forgiving about the more difficult ones. Getting a couple of films wrong does not mean that you will fail. In fact very few candidates get everything right. However, you will be marked down severely if you compromise patient safety (e.g. by suggesting a barium enema in a patient with toxic megacolon). At the time of publication, this component of the examination is still on hard copy (printed film), but the intention is to move to an electronic format in the near future. This is likely to occur when the exam is first held in the new RCR building, probably in Spring 2013.

Chapter 2

Our guide on how to pass the Final FRCR 2B

As with all professional examinations, this is a test of several facets of you as a candidate. You have to observe, think fast, show your knowledge and convey this either in written form or verbally.

RAPID REPORTING

In the past, when this component was on hard copy, there were several techniques which are now largely irrelevant. However, regardless of the format, a significant number of candidates seem to struggle with this section.

In the rapid reporting section of this book, we will show you examples of standard rapid reporting films. The key is to have (if you do not have already) a checklist of abnormalities that you search for on every type of film. Instead of providing practice rapid reporting examinations containing normal and abnormal films, we have only included the abnormal films, to show you what kind of abnormalities you can expect in the actual examination. These abnormal films have been compiled according to specific anatomical regions (e.g. abdomen, chest, facial bones, etc.). Some of the films have abnormalities at the edge of the film and in review areas. Remember that the abnormality is not always in the area intended to be examined, so do not forget to check for a pneumothorax in a shoulder X-ray, for example.

Another critical aspect of passing this section is to practise doing what were traditionally known as 'rapid reporting bags' under time pressure. One suggestion is to create mock examinations, building up a collection over time, and swapping them around among your colleagues. If there are six of you studying together, making up one each gives you six practice examinations to do!

As you begin to practise, it will be quite disconcerting at first how many cases you get wrong. You will find as an individual that you are either an 'undercaller' or an 'overcaller', and modify this appropriately. For example, if you are an overcaller, that extremely subtle rib notching is probably not real! Remember that in the examination, an error rate of 10% (3 wrong out of 30) still allows you to pass. Although contentious, if this is extrapolated to clinical practice, it is probably similar to the error rate of a working radiologist!

Finally, with regard to the way you approach the actual examination, one technique that works well and which we recommend is to move as rapidly as you can through the 30 cases. Cases that you have decided are abnormal are easy. If they are abnormal, they are abnormal. You can write it down and then forget about it. With practice, you can probably make this first pass through all of these cases in around 15–20 minutes. You can then spend the rest of your time going back over the 'normals', because these are the ones that you will want to spend more time on.

REPORTING SESSION

Completing six cases in 55 minutes is surprisingly stressful, and timing is the key here. Be strict!

It is better to give yourself 8 minutes per case and move on regardless, rather than write reams and reams on three cases, but run out of time for the rest – particularly if you have grossly misinterpreted the findings! Clearly, you are more likely to pass with the first option.

Although the RCR gives you an option as to how to lay out your answer, we would recommend bullet points rather than free text, as they make the information easier for the examiner to read. The easier it is to read, the less the examiner has to struggle to find the important (and hopefully correct) facts that you have written down, and the more points you will score.

Remember that the college guidance points out that you do not need to repeat the clinical information or give dates of each examination in your answer unless directly relevant. Similarly, in the case of MRI, you do not need to list each sequence. However, it is important to read the clinical information that is given, as it may be critical.

Write legibly and succinctly. In addition, the examiners will penalise you for incorrect statements or management decisions so, for example, don't write a huge list of unlikely differentials.

Do not forget to look at the scout image of a CT or MRI if included, as it often contains useful information. Try to be specific if you can (e.g. state which vertebral body that lesion is in), and don't forget incidental findings.

One technique that was useful when the examination was on film was to pick the ones with the fewest sheets of film/images first! They were usually quicker and easier cases, allowed you to work ahead of your time schedule and also gave you confidence! Whether this technique is applicable to an electronic format has yet to be seen.

ORAL EXAMINATION

Different people will give you different advice about how to approach the viva. Such advice may not only vary but even be contradictory. However, the key to success is to develop your own system for coping with different films and with the day itself. Most of the advice below is common sense, but it also incorporates the views of a recent FRCR examiner. Remember to conduct yourself in a professional manner at all times. Wear a suit, be polite and sound confident.

Preparation

The best way to study for this exam is to build up slowly. A period of 6–8 weeks is recommended. Be careful not to do too much. Some candidates report 'burning out' just before the exam. Several methods of studying are recommended (*see* Box 2.1).

- See as many films as possible.
- Undertake as many practice vivas (with consultants, senior trainees, etc.) as you can.
- If you can, study with others. It will get you used to speaking aloud, and you can test each other.
- Go on exam preparation courses. These will show you how others are preparing around the country, and will reassure you that the films you are seeing in your own institution are not that different to everyone else's!
- Study by using books.

Box 2.1 Different methods of studying

Of the above, the most important method is simply to see as many films as possible. Look through the collection of your institution or mentor, with permission of course. Ask consultants and senior trainees to viva you with their film collections. It will soon become obvious that the same cases appear time and time again. Make a note of these and target your (small amount) of reading to these 'standard' films. Use them as a basis for learning limited lists of differential diagnoses. There is no point in memorising a book of differential diagnoses from cover to cover. If you are not an outspoken individual, practise presenting cases out loud.

Note that studying by using books appears last on the list above. Keep this type of studying to a minimum. Do not be tempted to learn a standard text (e.g. Grainger & Allison, Sutton, etc.). Testing knowledge of obscure facts is not the point – that was done in the FRCR 2A! The viva is a test of observation, (safe) interpretation and communication of the facts.

However, as with all viva voce examinations, it is also unfortunately a test of how you present yourself. Someone who can talk about a difficult film intelligently will do better than someone who flounders, even if neither of them really has a clue. Remember that there will be films for which even the examiners don't know the real diagnosis.

There is of course some book work to be done. I would recommend using case-based books such as 'Case Review Series' or 'Aunt Minnie's' to familiarise yourself with the wide variety of pathology that our specialty encompasses. The only other book that you really need is a book of differential diagnoses. Keep reference books handy for things you want to look up in more depth, but only dip into them for a few key facts.

The actual examination

Walk into the room and smile! When you enter the room you will be greeted by the examiners, who will introduce themselves and address you by your candidate number, not your name. It is important that you appear relaxed and confident, even though you will almost certainly be feeling anything but. Sit forward in your chair and don't fidget. You will be a consultant soon, and you will be expected to behave like one. The examiners are looking for you to demonstrate your knowledge, so talk through your thought processes (talk as you look). They do not expect you to be an expert in liver MRI with 30 years' experience, but they want you to be the equivalent of a safe, competent third/fourth-year UK radiology trainee.

Listen to the examiner

Contrary to popular belief, the examiners *do* want you to pass. If you can demonstrate your knowledge and skills to them, this will make their task much more straightforward and pleasant. If they tell you something, it is generally to help you, not to trip you up. Listen to the examiner, as they will guide you. Some will ask 'Are you sure that is what it is?' to test the strength of your conviction. Others will say this because you have genuinely picked the wrong diagnosis. You have to be able to read the examiner as well as the films! Although some examiners may want you just to give the diagnosis if you know it, most would expect you to give a clear description of the findings before offering a diagnosis. *You won't know what is expected of you until you start*, but then you must interact with the examiner and work out quickly what they want from you. The best candidates often report that the exam felt more like a 'chat' than a 'grilling.'

Standard films

There are 'standard films' interspersed throughout this book. These are films that you should be able to talk about without actually having a film in front of you. They will become obvious as you prepare for the exam. Examples include multiple pulmonary nodules, lower zone lung fibrosis, and so on. As you read through the book, try to create a standard response for each of these films that you can use time and time again. You will find that after a while you don't actually need the film in front of you to regurgitate the response!

Presenting a film

As you describe each film, you will probably use phrases and expressions that you have thought about and included in your armoury. Some suggestions are listed below.

Useful phrases

- 'These are axial non-contrast CT images of the head of a … -year-old male.'
- 'In my normal practice I would look at previous films/control films/pre-contrast films …'
- 'The lesion appears to enhance, although I would normally confirm this with pre-contrast films.'
- 'I would compare this with previous films, looking for …'
- 'My usual system for looking at a CT abdomen is organ based. I am therefore now looking at the liver, spleen … (etc.).'
- 'I would consider X if the history indicated Y.'
- 'I can see no obvious abnormality, so will therefore check my review areas, which are …'
- 'I would arrange an MRI looking for … if … and might expect …'
- 'With symmetrical hydrocephalus, I am now looking for a colloid cyst/intraventricular blood …'
- 'I note the apparent density within the basal cisterns, which is thought to be due to compression, although I have considered SAH.'
- 'If the patient was unwell, I would consider …'
- 'The patient is clearly unwell, and I would immediately contact the clinican/local neurosurgical service.'
- 'I am not sure what this is, but would consider … and would take it further with …'
- 'In summary, … '

Phrases to avoid

- Do not say 'the obvious abnormality' – you may have missed the point of the film!
- Do not criticise the quality of the film. It may be the examiner's favourite film from their heady trainee days of 1980.

Finally, if you feel that you are on completely the wrong track, it is better to start again than to carry on talking rubbish. Take control of the situation and use turns of phrase such as 'Having reconsidered the findings/having now seen ..., I'd like to retract what I've said ...' to take the case forward.

Lists of differential diagnoses

Keep these short, and always give the most common and relevant ones first. I would suggest giving three or four, and then pausing. The examiner will prompt you for more obscure ones, or for the correct one, if they want more. However, make sure that you don't regurgitate lists straight from the book (easily done if you are desperately trying to remember a list you last looked at two months ago). You wouldn't put hypertrophic pyloric stenosis top of your list of causes for gastric outlet obstruction in a 70-year-old man when at work, so don't do it just because you're in an exam! Remember that it is often the case that 'unusual presentations of common disease are more likely than a common presentation of an unusual disease'.

The perfect film

The film goes up, you glance at it, and you have seen a hundred examples of this before. There are two methods of dealing with this film, but it is amazing how many candidates become confused. Some spend ages describing every tophus and every juxta-articular erosion when this isn't necessary. However, it must be reiterated that the right method should be found for every examiner. Try one method. If they frown, switch to another for subsequent films.

- Method 1: Don't waste time, but describe the findings quickly and succinctly, and then give the diagnosis. This will be the 'blurb' that you have practised time and time again. This is the preferred option.
- Method 2: It's an Aunt Minnie, so just say what it is (but try not to sound either elated or arrogant). Having given the diagnosis, you should probably go on to describe the findings that have led you to it. The film may well come down before you finish. However, the danger of giving your diagnosis too quickly is that it can unsettle the examiner who is not ready with their next case, and will lead to a difficult question, as they stall for time! Remember that real 'Aunt Minnies' such as osteopoikilosis are not favoured by examiners, as they are not discriminatory and are only occasionally encountered.

More information

With some films, you may feel that you need more information (e.g. exactly how ill the patient is). The best way to obtain this information is controversial. Some authors recommend that you ask the examiner directly. However, a better suggestion is to turn the question into an answer. For example, 'If the patient is septic I would consider ... but if not, then top of my differentials would be ...' The advantage of the second technique is that it shows your knowledge without the examiner having to ask, and it keeps you talking (and sounding intelligent) even if you aren't sure of the exact diagnosis.

Old films

Old films are important in routine practice and are therefore also important in the exam. Instead of asking 'Are there any old films?', which could easily elicit an unhelpful and show-stopping 'No', you could employ a similar tactic to that described above: 'If there were old films [pause and see if they are given to you, and if they are not, continue] ... I would expect to see ...'

Ending the film

Often you will describe the findings and give a diagnosis. The examiner will then engage you in a discussion. The problem for many candidates is ending the film. How does the examiner know that you have said all that you wanted to say? Petering out followed by silence is no good! You must end the film!

- You have made a decision. Stick by it confidently (even if you are wrong).
- If it has been a long description, you could say 'So, in summary ...'
- A good tip, at the end of every film, is to ask yourself 'What would I do next in real life?' For example:
  - 'This requires no follow-up'
  - 'This requires a repeat examination'
  - 'This requires urgent referral to Neurosurgery', etc.
- Finally, turn and look the examiner in the eye and let them know that you have finished.

The 'Help me, I have no idea' film

The film goes up, and you have no idea what it is. Keep calm. Don't panic. This is where you need a system and some stock phrases. It is not helpful to either you or the examiner for you to remain silent. Talk as you look. It will show the examiner that you have both a method of interpreting films and an underlying knowledge.

OK. You've employed some of your stock phrases, but the examiner is silent and you still have no idea. Are there any images that you have glossed over? Have you checked the scout images (on CT or MRI)? You may have been right so far, but is there a second or third abnormality?

If at the end of the day you are still stuck, and if all else fails, I would suggest that you sit back and say 'I'm sorry, but without further information I cannot take this film any further', then look the examiner in the eye! It is better to admit that you don't know than to keep digging a hole for yourself. It is also better to admit defeat so that you can move on quickly to the next film and gain credit for what you do know.

Section II

Chapter 1
Reporting session

Case bag 1

CASE 1.1

Age: 72 years	Gender: Male
Clinical problem: Back pain following a fall	
Images in exam case: Plain radiograph (4), CT (2)	

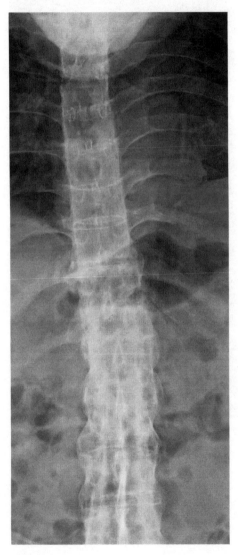

Figure 1a

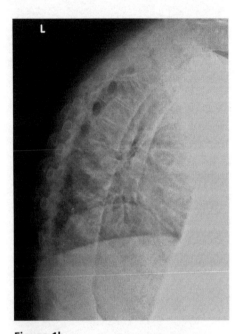

Figure 1b

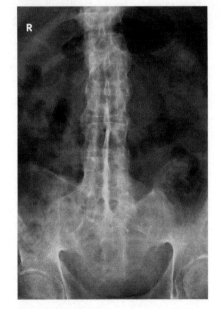

Figure 1c

Figure 1d

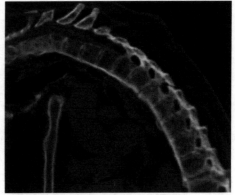

Figure 1e

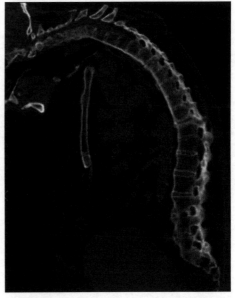

Figure 1f

FINDINGS

1. X-ray thoracolumbar spine:
   a. Marginal syndesmophytes
   b. Ossification of the interspinous ligament – 'dagger' sign
   c. Ossification of the anterior longitudinal ligament
   d. Fusion of both sacroiliac joints
   e. Fracture through mid-thoracic intervertebral disc with retrolisthesis of superior vertebra.
2. CT whole spine:
   a. Ossification of anterior longitudinal ligament
   b. Fusion of multiple facet joints
   c. Severe cervicothoracic kyphosis
   d. Fracture line starting at D5/6 intervertebral disc and extending into the posterosuperior body of D6 and D6/7 facet joints
   e. Mild retrolisthesis of D5 over D6
   f. Widened lucent line through D10/11 disc space and facet joints with adjacent reactive sclerosis
   g. Distended urinary bladder.

DIAGNOSIS

1. Ankylosing spondylitis, acute fracture through D5/6 extending through the posterior elements. This is an unstable fracture as all three vertebral columns are disrupted.
2. Pseudoarthrosis D10/11, most likely secondary to non-union of an old fracture.

FURTHER INVESTIGATIONS AND MANAGEMENT

1. Urgent neurosurgical referral, as the fracture is unstable.
2. If there are signs of cord compression, MRI may be necessary to look for cord injury or spinal extra-axial haematoma.

FURTHER INFORMATION

Ankylosing spondylitis is a regular feature of the FRCR 2B examination, either as a written case or in the viva. The scenarios involved could be bilateral symmetrical sacroiliac joint erosion, sclerosis or fusion, erosion of the anterosuperior corner of the vertebra on lateral radiograph (Romanus sign), sclerosis of the anterosuperior corner and periostitis of the waist giving rise to vertebral 'squaring', syndesmophyte formation leading to 'bamboo spine', intervertebral disc calcification, ossification of the anterior longitudinal, posterior longitudinal, interspinous and supraspinous ligaments, kyphosis and facet joint fusion. Other skeletal features include erosions of the symphysis pubis and ischial tuberosities, asymmetrical erosive oligoarthritis, atlanto-axial dislocation and osteoporosis. In a traumatic setting, the fracture line may run through the intervertebral disc space right through into the posterior elements, and may be missed if one is not vigilant. Clinically occult fractures can also occur, leading to mobile non-union (pseudoarthrosis) – the so-called Anderson lesion.

CASE 1.2

Age: 63 years	Gender: Male
Clinical problem: History of rectal carcinoma. Abnormal findings on staging CT	
Images in exam case: CT (1), MRI (5)	

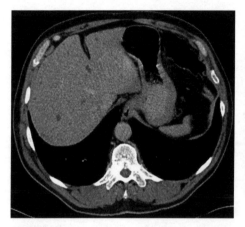

Figure 2a

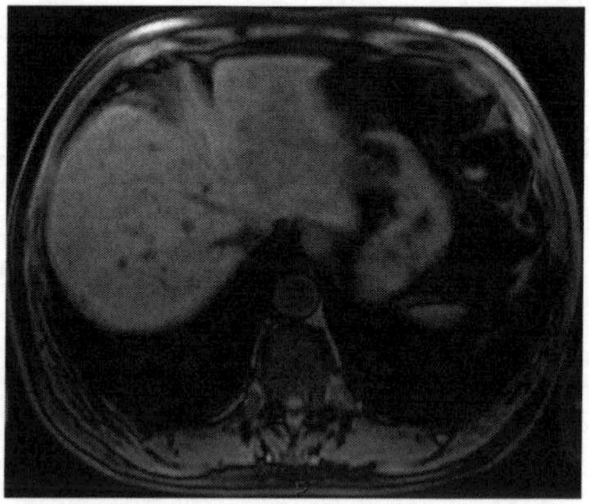

Figure 2b

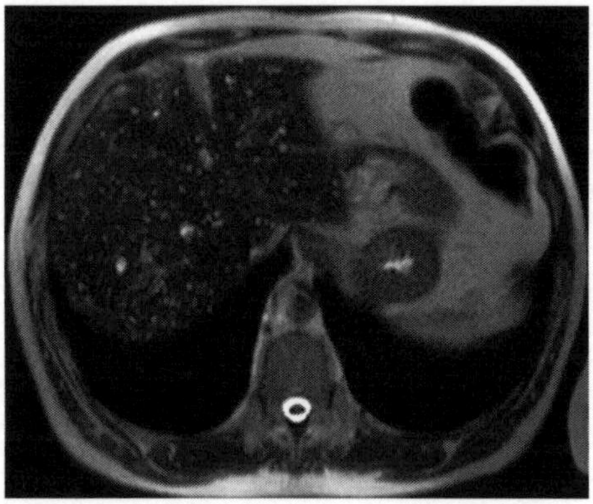

Figure 2c

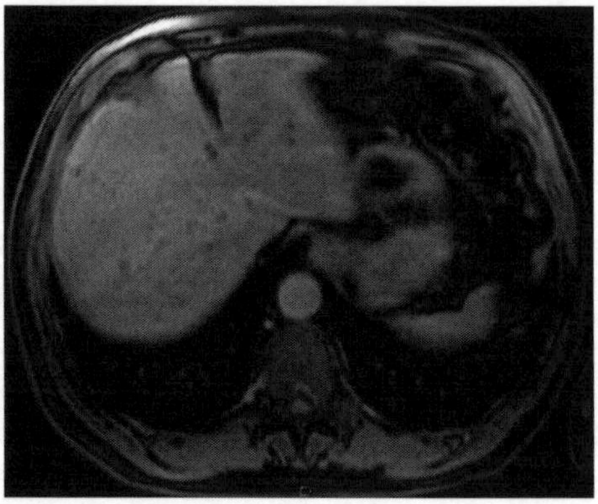

Figure 2d (arterial phase)

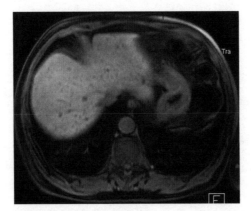

Figure 2e (venous phase)

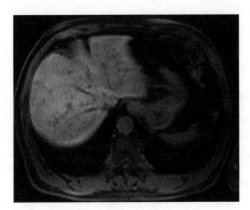

Figure 2f (15-minute delayed)

FINDINGS

1. CT abdomen: multiple small low-attenuation liver lesions in both lobes of the liver.
2. Pre-contrast T1-weighted image: multiple small low-signal liver lesions.
3. T2-weighted image: Innumerable small high-signal lesions throughout the liver.
4. Arterial, venous and 15-minute delayed phase post-contrast T1-weighted images: no enhancement of the liver lesions.

INTERPRETATION

Innumerable, uniform, small cystic lesions of the liver.

MAIN DIAGNOSIS

Multiple biliary hamartomas.

DIFFERENTIAL DIAGNOSIS

1. Multiple metastases. However, the uniform size and signal intensity and absence of post-contrast enhancement are features that argue against the diagnosis of metastases.
2. Multiple microabscesses from candida infection. However, the patients are generally immunocompromised, and both the liver and spleen are involved. In immunocompetent patients, candida microabscesses show mural enhancement.

FURTHER INVESTIGATIONS AND MANAGEMENT

Biliary hamartomas are benign, and no further treatment is required.

FURTHER INFORMATION

Biliary hamartomas, also called von Meyenburg complexes, are thought to arise from embryonic bile ducts that fail to involute. The lesions are common (they are present in approximately 3% of the population), and may be solitary or multiple. They are generally less than 1 cm in diameter, uniform and well defined. Most of them do not enhance, but some lesions may show rim enhancement due to compressed hepatic parenchyma. The potential pitfall is to call these lesions metastases because of this apparent rim enhancement. Although enhancement of metastases often progresses centrally, enhancement in biliary hamartomas does not progress centrally.

CASE 1.3

Age: 68 years	Gender: Male
Clinical problem: Occipital headache and vomiting	
Images in exam case: CT (1), CT angiogram (3)	

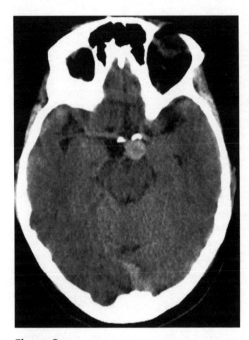

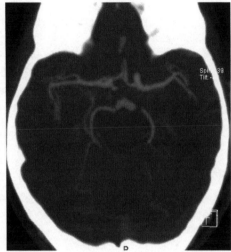

Figure 3b

Figure 3a

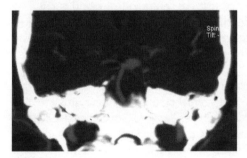

Figure 3c

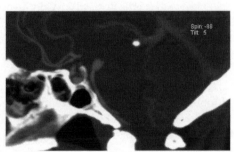

Figure 3d

FINDINGS

1. Non-contrast CT brain:
   a. Well-defined rounded hyperattenuating mass in the suprasellar cistern, slightly towards the left of the midline
   b. A hint of low attenuation at the centre of the mass
   c. Adjacent M1 segments of the middle cerebral arteries are calcified on both sides
   d. No mass effect and no adjacent parenchymal oedema
   e. No subarachnoid haemorrhage.
2. CT angiogram:
   a. Lobulated oval enhancing mass superiorly and to the left of the basilar artery
   b. Neck of the mass arising from the basilar artery tip.

DIAGNOSIS

Large berry aneurysm at the tip of the basilar artery.

FURTHER MANAGEMENT

1. As the patient is symptomatic with headache and vomiting, immediate referral to neurointerventional radiologists for potential coiling of the aneurysm.
2. A thorough search for other aneuryms, as multiple aneurysms can coexist.

FURTHER INFORMATION

Berry aneurysms occur in approximately 3–4% of the population, and in 20–30% of cases these are multiple. Aneurysms can present as subarachnoid, intraparenchymal and intra-ventricular haemorrhage. Rarely, a ruptured aneurysm can give rise to a subdural haemor-rhage. The annual risk of rupture for aneurysms < 10 mm in diameter is 0.1%, and for aneurysms > 10 mm it is 0.5%. On CT the greatest concentration of blood is close to the aneurysm that has bled. Blood in the interhemispheric cistern and lateral ventricle suggests anterior communicating artery aneurysm, blood in the Sylvian fissure suggests middle cerebral artery aneurysm, and blood in the fourth ventricle suggests posterior infe-rior cerebellar artery aneurysm.

Giant aneurysms, which are > 2.5 cm in diameter, account for 5% of cases. Their risk of rupture is higher (approximately 6% in the first year of diagnosis). Aneurysms can also present with mass effect giving rise to cranial nerve palsies – painful 3rd cranial nerve palsy with posterior communicating artery aneurysm, 6th cranial nerve palsy with aneurysm in the cavernous sinus and visual field defects from supraclinoid carotid or anterior cerebral artery aneurysm.

There are a number of conditions associated with intracranial aneurysms. The impor-tant ones are autosomal dominant polycystic kidney disease (ADPKD), coarctation of the aorta, fibromuscular dysplasia, Marfan's syndrome, neurofibromatosis type 1 and Takaya-su's disease (an exhaustive list can be found in *Neuroradiology: the Requisites*, 2nd edi-tion, by RI Grossman and DM Yousem).

CASE 1.4

Age: 47 years	Gender: Female
Clinical problem: Vomiting and severe epigastric pain	
Images in exam case: Plain radiograph (1), CT (3), contrast series (2)	

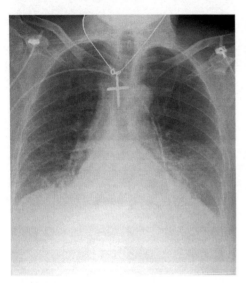

Figure 4a

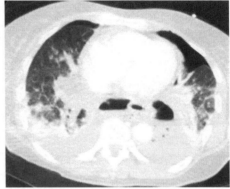

Figure 4b

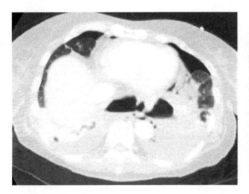

Figure 4c

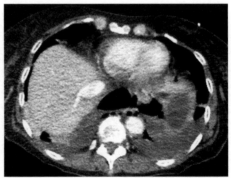

Figure 4d

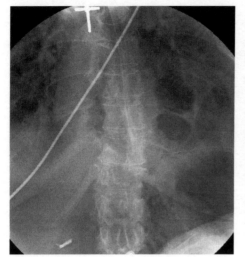 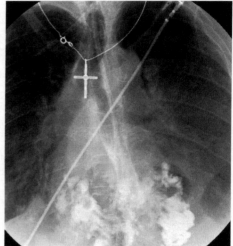

Figure 4e   **Figure 4f**

FINDINGS

1. Chest X-ray:
   a. ECG leads and oxygen tubing
   b. Gas projected behind the heart
   c. Blunting of both costophrenic angles, most probably from bilateral pleural effusions
   d. No free gas under the diaphragm.
2. CT thorax:
   a. Bilateral hydropneumothoraces and basal atelectases
   b. Pockets of gas within the mediastinum, particularly around the oesophagus and prevertebral region.
3. Contrast swallow examination:
   a. Leakage of contrast outwith the distal oesophagus on either side
   b. NG tube *in situ* with the tip below the level of the diaphragm
   c. Surgical clip from previous cholecystectomy.

DIAGNOSIS

Perforation of the distal oesophagus (Boerhaave syndrome) causing pneumomediastinum and bilateral hydropneumothoraces.

FURTHER MANAGEMENT

Immediate surgical referral for emergency surgery.

FURTHER INFORMATION

Spontaneous oesophageal perforation, also called Boerhaave syndrome, results from excessive forceful vomiting. Severe chest pain occurs, followed by rapid progression to mediastinitis as oesophageal contents enter the mediastinum. Delay in diagnosis is a major factor contributing to high mortality. Usually there is a large defect in the distal oesophagus approximately 2–3 cm proximal to the gastro-oesophageal junction. The defect usually occurs on the left side. In this case, rupture has occurred on either side of the distal oesophagus. Pneumomediastinum, pneumothorax, pleural effusion/hydropneumothorax, surgical emphysema and widened mediastinum are the main radiological findings.

CASE 1.5

Age: 70 years	Gender: Male
Clinical problem: Epigastric pain and weight loss	
Images in exam case: CT (2), MRI (3)	

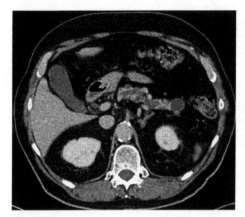

Figure 5a

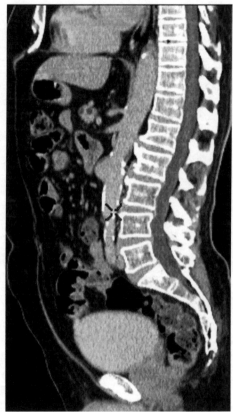

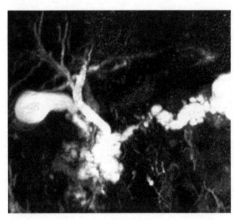

Figure 5c

Figure 5b

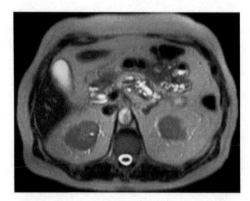

Figure 5d

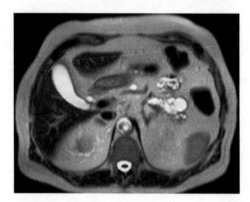

Figure 5e

FINDINGS

1. CT abdomen:
   a. Dilated main pancreatic duct with multiple cystic dilated side branches
   b. Atrophic pancreas
   c. No evidence of solid pancreatic mass
   d. No pancreatic calcification or ductal calculi
   e. Focal abdominal aortic aneurysm
   f. Degenerative changes of the lumbar spine.
2. MRI: Dilated pancreatic duct with multiple cystic dilated side branches throughout the pancreas.

MAIN DIAGNOSIS

1. Intraductal papillary mucinous tumour (IPMT) of pancreas.
2. Abdominal aortic aneurysm.

DIFFERENTIAL DIAGNOSIS

Chronic pancreatitis. However, this is unlikely as there is no pancreatic calcification.

FURTHER INVESTIGATIONS AND MANAGEMENT

1. Surgical referral, as these tumours are considered to be premalignant.
2. EUS may be helpful for distinguishing invasive from non-invasive lesions.

FURTHER INFORMATION

IPMTs of pancreas are mucin-producing tumours of the pancreatic ducts. They have low malignant potential, grow slowly and rarely metastasise. These tumours are more common in men, and epigastric pain, weight loss, diabetes and sometimes a palpable mass are the presenting problems. Mucin plugs obstruct the main or side ducts, causing ductal dilatation. Two types of IPMT of pancreas have been described, namely main duct and side duct types. The side duct type has a cystic mass that is either unilocular or consists of a cluster of small cysts, and the main duct type has diffuse pancreatic ductal dilatation with atrophy of the pancreatic parenchyma. On ERCP, large amounts of mucin are seen exuding from the papilla. As all main duct type IPMTs are considered to be premalignant, resection is the treatment of choice.

CASE 1.6

Age: 30 years	Gender: Female
Clinical problem: Dry cough and night sweats	
Images in exam case: Plain radiograph (1), CT (4)	

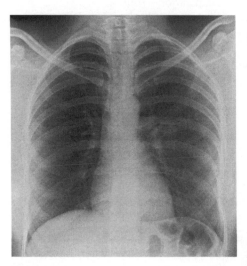

Figure 6a

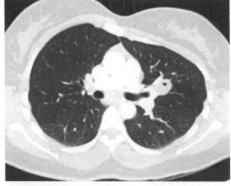

Figure 6c

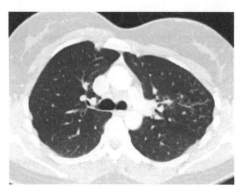

Figure 6b

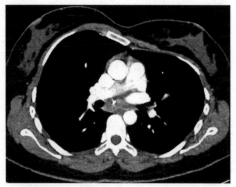

Figure 6d

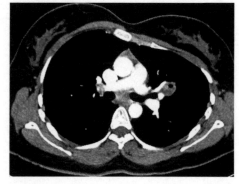

Figure 6e

FINDINGS

1. Chest X-ray: Well-defined soft tissue mass, approximately 3 cm in diameter, adjacent to the left hilum.
2. CT thorax:
   a. Well-defined, non-spiculated, cavitating mass adjacent to the left hilum
   b. 'Tree-in-bud' nodularity in the left upper lobe
   c. Enlarged subcarinal lymph node with calcification within it.

MAIN DIAGNOSIS

Cavitating pulmonary tuberculosis with endobronchial spread and mediastinal lymph node enlargement.

DIFFERENTIAL DIAGNOSIS

Cavitating bronchogenic carcinoma. However, this is less likely as the patient is relatively young.

FURTHER INVESTIGATIONS AND MANAGEMENT

1. Urgent respiratory referral.
2. Sputum culture for tuberculosis. Bronchoscopy for washings and biopsy if necessary.

FURTHER INFORMATION

Primary tuberculosis can present as consolidation like any other bacterial pneumonia. Pleural effusion and mediastinal lymph node enlargement may occur. The primary complex is a subpleural focus of infection (Gohn focus) in combination with regional (hilar) lymph node enlargement. When an infected focus erodes into the tracheobronchial tree, endobronchial spread occurs and is seen as 'tree-in-bud' nodularity. Besides the lungs, primary tuberculosis can occur in the intestines, tonsils and skin. Primary tuberculosis can either heal with calcification or spread via haematogenous or lymphatic routes. Rapid venous dissemination causes miliary tuberculosis. Disseminated tuberculosis can also affect the meninges, bones, genitourinary tract, liver and spleen. Post-primary or reactivation tuberculosis presents as consolidation and cavitation, particularly in the upper lobes or apical segments of the lower lobes.

Case bag 2

CASE 2.1

Age: 39 years	Gender: Male
Clinical problem: Left-sided weakness and right miosis and ptosis	
Images in exam case: CT (1), MRI (5), CT angiogram (2)	

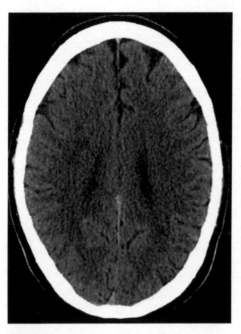

Figure 7a

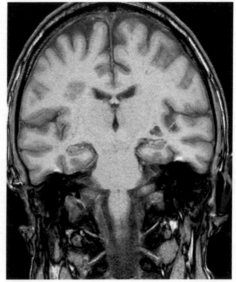

Figure 7b

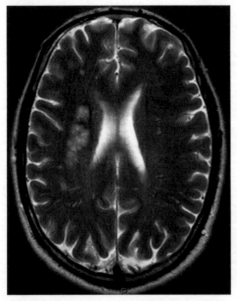

Figure 7c

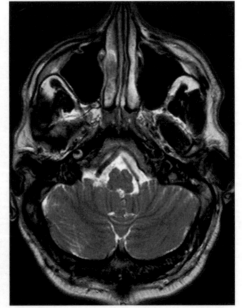

Figure 7d

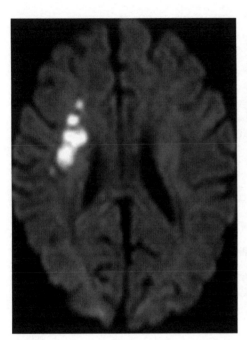

Figure 7e

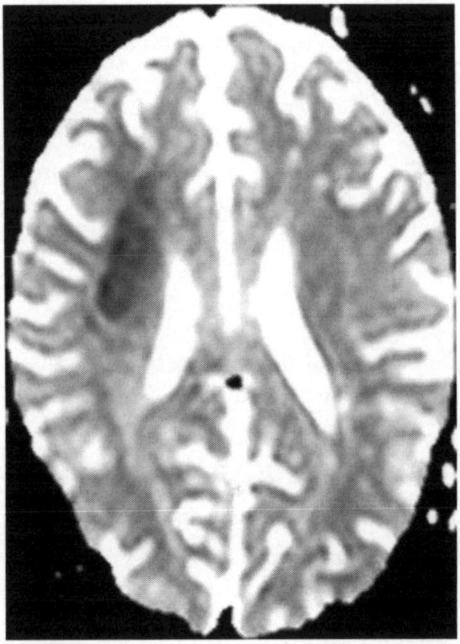

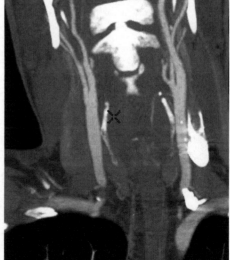

Figure 7f

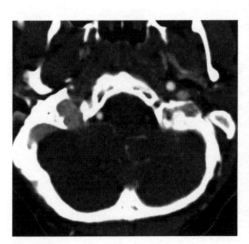

Figure 7g

Figure 7h

FINDINGS

1. CT brain: Low attenuation within the right internal border zone territory.
2. T1 coronal MRI: Low signal in the right internal border zone territory.
3. T2 axial MRI:
    a. Corresponding high signal
    b. High-signal intramural thrombus within the right internal carotid artery with eccentric flow void.
4. DWI and ADC maps: High signal on DWI with corresponding low signal on ADC map in the right internal border zone territory consistent with acute infarction.
5. CT angiography:
    a. Expanded right internal carotid artery with mural thrombus and markedly attenuated eccentric right lumen just as it enters the carotid canal
    b. Coronal reformatted MIP CTA: narrowing of the right internal carotid artery above the level of the C2 transverse process.

DIAGNOSIS

Right internal carotid artery dissection causing right internal border zone territory infarction and Horner's syndrome.

FURTHER INVESTIGATIONS AND MANAGEMENT

1. Neurology referral with a view to anticoagulation.
2. Assessment for risk factors of spontaneous dissection (e.g. hypertension).

FURTHER INFORMATION

Vascular dissection is an important cause of stroke in young patients, particularly in individuals with no apparent risk factors. Patients with extracranial arterial dissection can present with neck/facial pain, headache, Horner's syndrome, cranial nerve palsies and symptoms of ischaemia. Ischaemic symptoms can be somewhat delayed in extracranial dissection, whereas in intracranial dissection these symptoms progress quickly. Fibromuscular disease, Ehlers–Danlos syndrome, hypertension, Marfan syndrome and autosomal dominant polycystic kidney disease are some of the predisposing conditions for arterial dissection.

Extracranial dissections cause stroke and TIAs, particularly affecting the border zone territories, due to compromised blood supply. Stroke and TIAs can also result from distal embolic phenomena secondary to these extracranial dissections. Fat-suppressed T1-weighted axial images are excellent for visualisation of arterial dissection. Subintimal haematoma is visualised as an eccentric high signal with a narrowed (fried-egg sign) or completely absent flow void in the affected segment.

CASE 2.2

Age: 28 years	Gender: Female
Clinical problem: Shortness of breath (the patient is a smoker)	
Images in exam case: Plain radiograph (1), CT (3)	

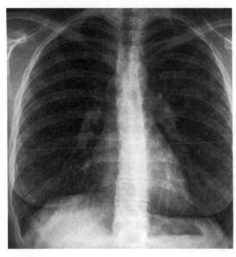

Figure 8a

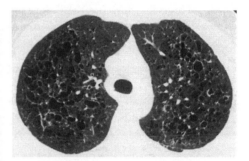

Figure 8b

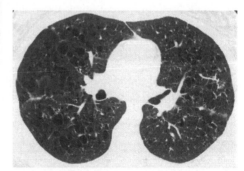

Figure 8c

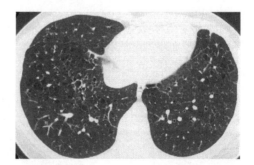

Figure 8d

FINDINGS

1. Chest X-ray:
   a. Bilateral symmetrical coarse reticular opacification
   b. Normal lung volumes.
2. HRCT thorax:
   a. Multiple variable-sized, thin-walled pulmonary cysts – some are of bizarre irregular shape
   b. Cysts are more predominant in the upper and mid zones than at the base
   c. The anterior aspects of the middle lobe and lingula are spared
   d. Intervening lung parenchyma is normal.

MAIN DIAGNOSIS

Pulmonary Langerhans cell histiocytosis (LCH). Although the condition is more common in males, the distribution and shape of the cysts and history of smoking support this diagnosis.

DIFFERENTIAL DIAGNOSIS

1. Lymphangiomyomatosis (LAM) – cysts are generally round, uniform and diffuse.
2. Lymphoid interstitial pneumonitis (LIP) – cysts are less numerous than in LCH or LAM.

FURTHER INVESTIGATIONS AND MANAGEMENT

1. Cessation of smoking.
2. Respiratory referral for potential chemotherapy.

FURTHER INFORMATION

LCH and LAM must be suspected if there is evidence of interstitial lung disease with normal or increased lung volumes on plain radiographs. LAM occurs mainly in females of childbearing age, and is associated with tuberous sclerosis. Chylous pleural effusion may be present. Cysts are generally round, uniform and diffuse. In LCH, the costophrenic angles may be spared and the cysts are of irregular configuration. There may be small irregular peribronchial nodules. LCH is common in heavy cigarette smokers, and is more common in males than in females, with a 4:1 male:female ratio. Smoking cessation may result in a significant improvement.

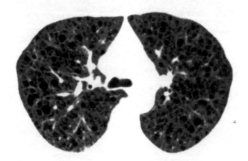

Figure 8e: LAM (note uniformity of cysts).

CASE 2.3

Age: 53 years	Gender: Male
Clinical problem: Night sweats and abnormal LFTs	
Images in exam case: US (1), CT (4), MRI (5)	

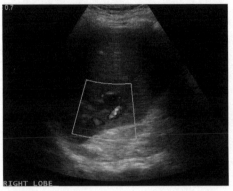

Figure 9a

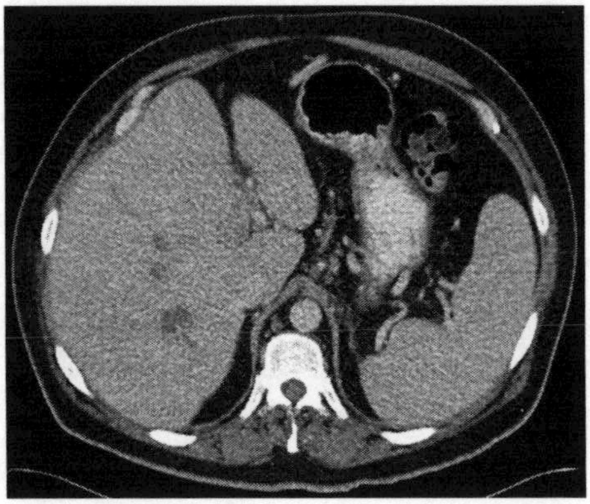

Figure 9b

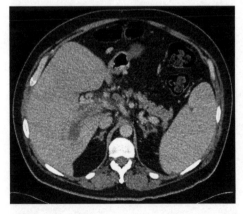

Figure 9c

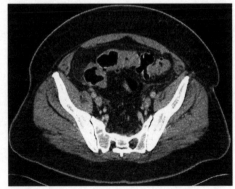

Figure 9d

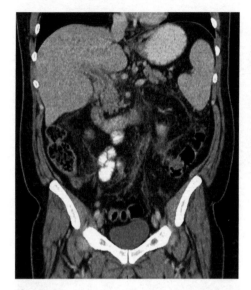

Figure 9e

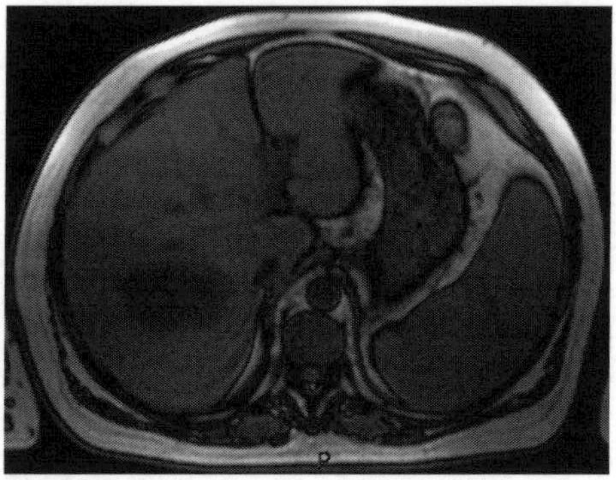

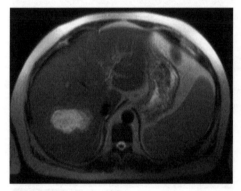

Figure 9f

Figure 9g

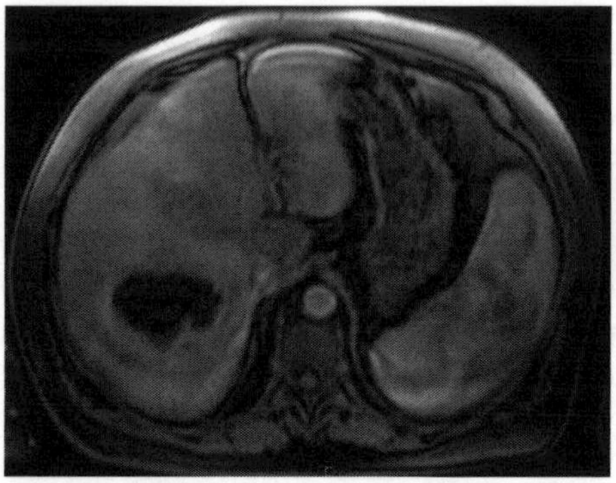

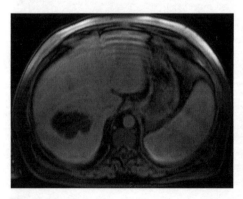

Figure 9i

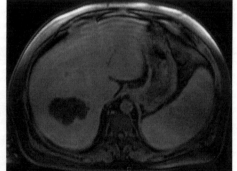

Figure 9h

Figure 9j

FINDINGS

1. US liver:
   a. Hypoechoic region within the right lobe of liver
   b. No Doppler signal within the lesion.
2. CT abdomen:
   a. Ill-defined low-attenuation lesion within the right lobe of liver
   b. Portal vein thrombosis extending into the right branch
   c. Thrombosis of the inferior mesenteric vein with fatty stranding surrounding the vein
   d. Diverticular disease of the sigmoid colon with evidence of wall thickening
   e. Bulky spleen.
3. MRI liver:
   a. T1 hypointense lesion within the right lobe of liver
   b. The lesion is hyperintense on T2 and has a thick irregular capsule
   c. Minimal enhancement of the capsule in arterial phase
   d. No central enhancement of the lesion in arterial, venous or delayed phases.

MAIN DIAGNOSIS

Liver abscess of the right lobe of liver secondary to sigmoid diverticulitis causing IMV and portal pyaemia.

DIFFERENTIAL DIAGNOSIS

Liver metastasis with a large central necrotic component. However, the presence of diverticulitis, and IMV and portal vein thrombosis, favour the diagnosis of liver abscess.

FURTHER INVESTIGATIONS AND MANAGEMENT

1. Ultrasound-guided aspiration.
2. Culture and cytology of aspirate.
3. Gastroenterology referral for appropriate antibiotic treatment.

FURTHER INFORMATION

Pyogenic liver abscesses are frequently associated with portal vein thrombosis. Abscesses may also show a perilesional hyperaemic inflammatory response in early post-contrast images. Internal septations, fluid-fluid level due to layering of proteinaceous debris and locules of gas are other features that may be present. Sometimes multiple pyogenic liver abscesses can occur as a cluster of lesions. Metastasis with a necrotic centre may mimic an abscess because of an enhancing rim.

CASE 2.4

Age: 82 years	Gender: Male
Clinical problem: Bone pain	
Images in exam case: Plain radiograph (2), Radionuclide scan (1)	

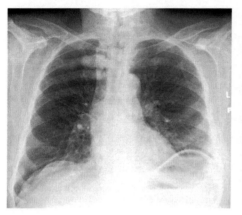

Figure 10a

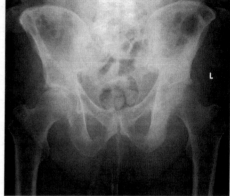

Figure 10b

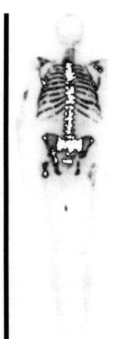

Figure 10c

FINDINGS

1. Chest X-ray:
   a. Sclerotic expansile lesions of the right 4th and 5th ribs in the posterior aspect
   b. No focal lung lesion.
2. X-ray pelvis: Sclerosis of the left iliac bone and inferior pubic ramus.
3. Radionuclide bone scan:
   a. Increased uptake throughout the ribs, vertebral bodies and pelvic girdle
   b. High sternal uptake – 'tie sign'
   c. No uptake within the kidneys
   d. Urinary catheter *in situ*.

INTERPRETATION

Extensive sclerotic bone metastases with 'superscan' appearance in radionuclide bone scan. The presence of an indwelling catheter suggests urinary outflow obstruction.

MAIN DIAGNOSIS

Prostate cancer with diffuse bone metastases.

DIFFERENTIAL DIAGNOSIS

1. Other causes of sclerotic metastases (e.g. carcinoma of lung, bladder, colon or stomach).
2. Other causes of superscan (e.g. renal osteodystrophy, hyperparathyroidism – these are less likely as there is no subperiosteal resorption, rugger-jersey spine or brown tumours).

FURTHER INVESTIGATIONS AND MANAGEMENT

1. Determine whether there is a known history of prostate cancer.
2. Recommend measurement of prostate-specific antigen (PSA).
3. Urology referral.

FURTHER INFORMATION

Superscan occurs when there is diffuse high bone uptake of the radionuclide with diminished soft tissue and renal activity. Although there is non-visualisation of the kidneys, the bladder is often well visualised (absent kidney sign). The sternum and costochondral junctions may show high uptake. The causes are diffuse bone metastases (e.g. from prostate and breast cancer), metabolic bone diseases (e.g. hyperparathyroidism, renal osteodystrophy, osteomalacia, Paget's disease) or myeloproliferative disorders. In some cases, the uptake is so diffuse that it can be mistaken for normal.

CASE 2.5

Age: 81 years	Gender: Female
Clinical problem: Pelvic mass	
Images in exam case: MRI (3)	

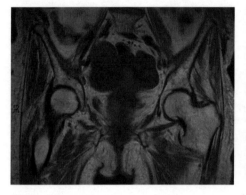

Figure 11a

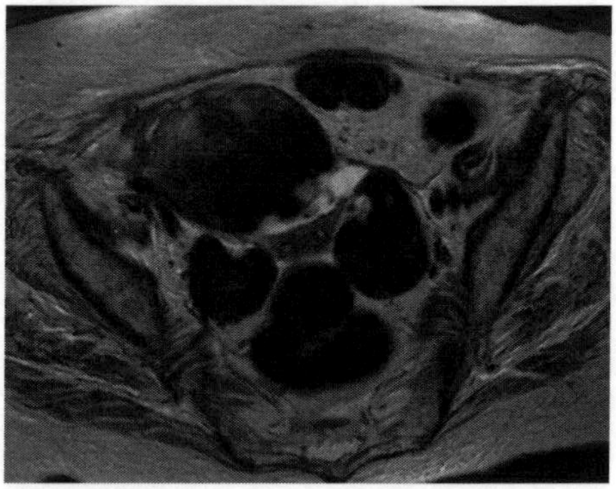

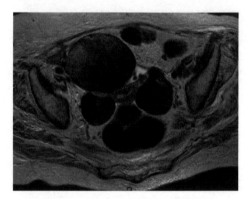

Figure 11b

Figure 11c

FINDINGS

1. T1 coronal:
   a. Bilateral well-defined lobulated low-signal adnexal masses.
2. T2 axial:
   a. Large rounded low-signal adnexal masses – one on the left and two on the right – which appear to arise from the ovaries
   b. Compressed residual right ovarian tissue
   c. Normal appearance of the uterus
   d. Trace of pelvic free fluid.

DIAGNOSIS

Bilateral ovarian fibroma/thecoma.

FURTHER INVESTIGATIONS AND MANAGEMENT

Gynaecological referral.

FURTHER INFORMATION

Ovarian fibromas/thecomas are the most common benign solid ovarian tumours. Histologically, fibromas and thecomas can overlap, hence the term fibrothecoma. These are benign ovarian neoplasms of sex cord–stromal origin. Thecomas can secrete oestrogen, so these patients are at risk of development of endometrial hyperplasia and carcinoma. Meigs' syndrome is a combination of ovarian fibroma with ascites and right pleural effusion. On MRI, ovarian fibrothecomas are hypointense on both T1- and T2-weighted images – similar to pedunculated fibroids – and it is thus sometimes difficult to be certain. Compressed ovarian tissue surrounding an ovarian mass may be visualised with ovarian fibrothecomas.

CASE 2.6

Age: 46 years	Gender: Male
Clinical problem: Abdominal discomfort	
Images in exam case: Plain radiograph (2), MRI (3)	

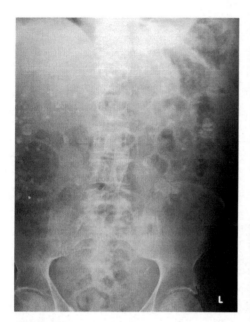

Figure 12a

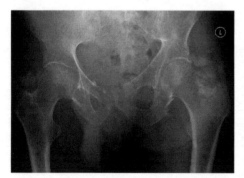

Figure 12b

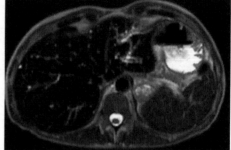

Figure 12c

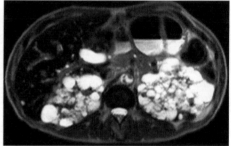

Figure 12d

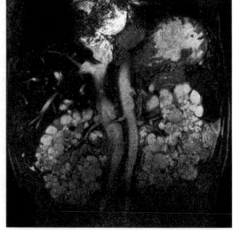

Figure 12e

FINDINGS

1. X-ray abdomen:
   a. Numerous rounded calcific densities projected over the lumbar region bilaterally
   b. Calcified distal abdominal aorta.
2. X-ray pelvis:
   a. Large lobulated soft tissue calcifications overlying both hip joints.
3. MRI liver – T2-weighted images:
   a. Generalised low signal in both liver and spleen
   b. Multiple small high-signal rounded areas throughout the liver
   c. Enlarged kidneys with innumerable rounded high-signal areas throughout both kidneys
   d. No normal intervening renal tissue.

MAIN DIAGNOSIS

1. Autosomal dominant polycystic kidney disease with multiple liver cysts.
2. Hepatosplenic haemosiderosis, most probably from multiple blood transfusions.
3. Soft tissue calcification, probably due to secondary hyperthyroidism.

DIFFERENTIAL DIAGNOSIS

Acquired cystic renal disease. However, as this condition is restricted to the kidneys, the presence of hepatic cysts argues against this diagnosis.

FURTHER INVESTIGATIONS AND MANAGEMENT

1. Nephrology follow-up with regard to monitoring renal function, control of hypertension, treatment of UTIs and renal replacement therapy for end-stage renal failure.

FURTHER INFORMATION

Autosomal dominant polycystic kidney disease (ADPCKD) has 100% penetrance, and 85% of cases are due to a mutation on chromosome 16, while 15% are due to a mutation on chromosome 4. Hypertension, cerebral aneurysms, aortic aneurysm, aortic dissection and valvular heart diseases can be associated with ADPCKD.

Renal tubular ectasia and hepatic fibrosis are features of autosomal recessive polycystic kidney disease (ARPCKD). This condition may present during the antenatal period, in infancy or in early childhood. The kidneys are enlarged and echogenic on ultrasound, and may have tiny cysts. The less severe the renal disease, the worse is the hepatic fibrosis.

Acquired cystic renal disease occurs in any form of end-stage renal disease, particularly if the patient has been on long-standing haemodialysis or peritoneal dialysis. The appearance of the kidneys can mimic autosomal dominant polycystic kidney disease (ADPKD). As the condition is restricted to the kidneys, the presence of cysts in the liver and pancreas favours the diagnosis of ADPKD.

Case bag 3

CASE 3.1

Age: 63 years	Gender: Female
Clinical problem: Headache, confusion and expressive dysphasia	
Images in exam case: CT (2), MRI (6)	

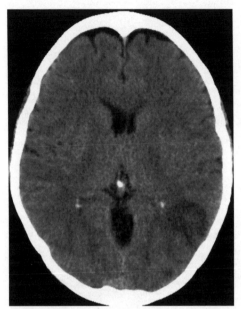

Figure 13a

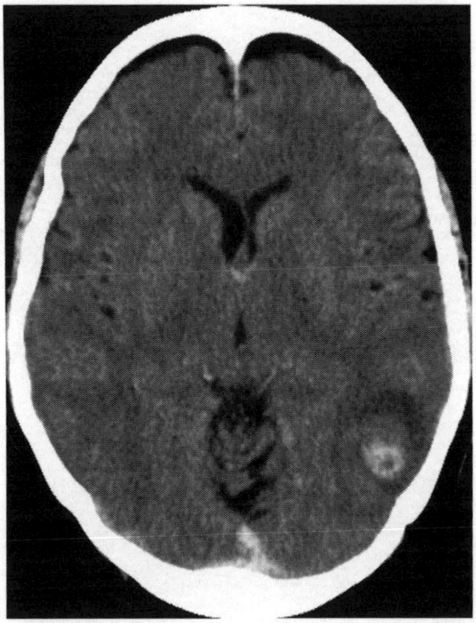

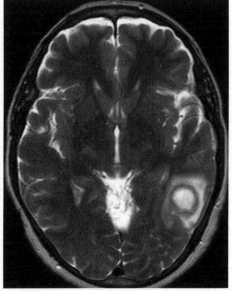

Figure 13b

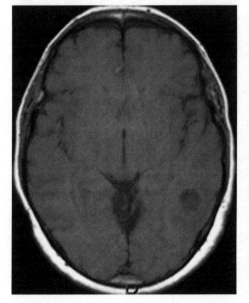

Figure 13c

Figure 13d

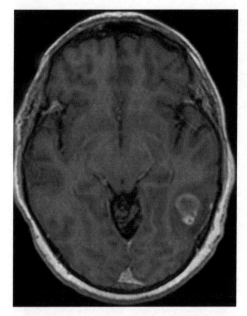

Figure 13e

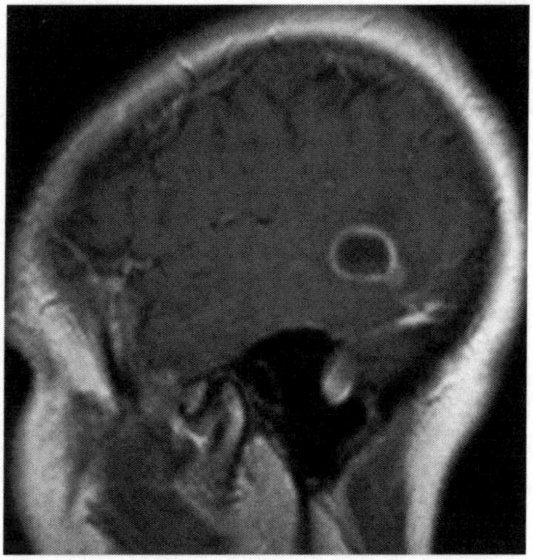

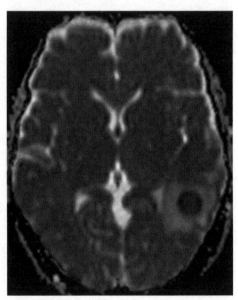

Figure 13f

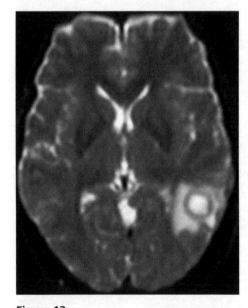

Figure 13g

Figure 13h

FINDINGS

1. Post-contrast CT brain:
   a. Ring-enhancing mass in the left parietotemporal region, approximately 2.5 cm in diameter
   b. Surrounding white matter oedema
   c. Mass effect causing local sulcal effacement.
2. T1-weighted MRI:
   a. The lesion has a central low signal and is surrounded by low-signal oedema.
3. T2-weighted MRI:
   a. The lesion has a high signal at the centre and is surrounded by a low-signal rim
   b. Surrounding high-signal oedema
   c. Local sulcal effacement and minimal effacement of the left lateral ventricle.
4. Post-contrast T1 images:
   a. Ring enhancement of the lesion
   b. Uniform thin wall
   c. Tiny daughter lesion abutting it posteriorly.
5. DWI and ADC map:
   a. The lesion is high signal on DWI and low signal on the ADC map, consistent with diffusion restriction.

INTERPRETATION

Left parietotemporal ring-enhancing mass that restricts diffusion.

MAIN DIAGNOSIS

Left parietotemporal brain abscess.

DIFFERENTIAL DIAGNOSIS

Necrotic primary or metastatic tumour, but these generally do not restrict diffusion.

FURTHER INVESTIGATIONS AND MANAGEMENT

Urgent referral to neurosurgery unit.

FURTHER INFORMATION

Brain abscesses can occur secondary to haematogenous seeding or from direct extension from adjacent infection (e.g. sinusitis, otitis media, etc.). Abscesses secondary to haematogenous seeding are at the grey–white matter junction, generally in the MCA distribution. Abscesses restrict diffusion due to high protein content and cellularity within the abscess cavity. Tiny daughter lesions also support the diagnosis, although these can also occur with gliomas. The abscess wall is generally smooth on the outside and irregular on the inside, and the wall can be thicker on the grey matter side and thinner on the white matter side. As a result, abscesses can rupture into ventricles, inciting ventriculitis.

CASE 3.2

Age: 52 years	Gender: Female
Clinical problem: Collapse	
Images in exam case: CT (1), MIBG scan (2)	

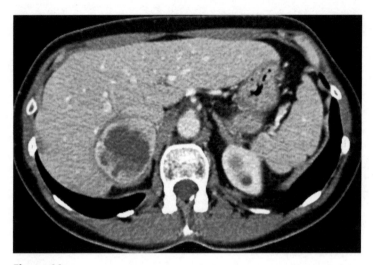

Figure 14a

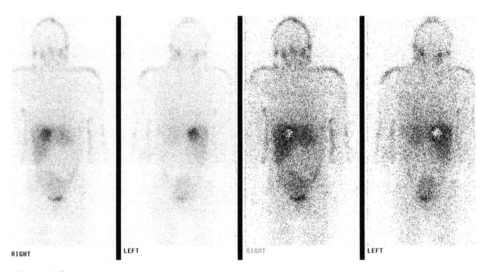

RIGHT   LEFT   RIGHT   LEFT

Figure 14b

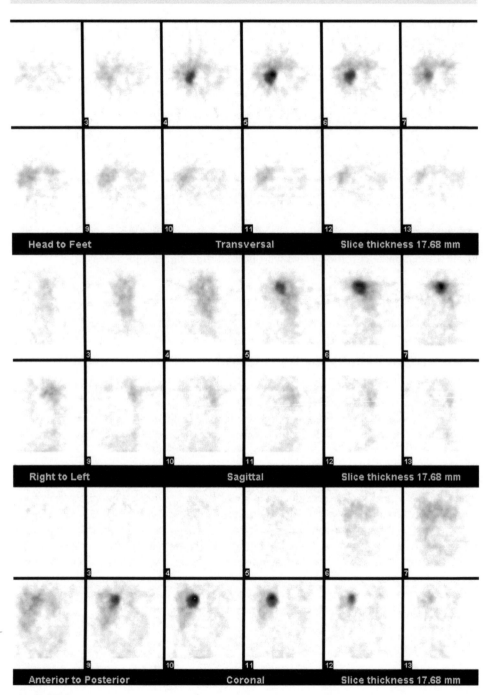

Figure 14c

FINDINGS

1. CT abdomen:
   a. Large enhancing rounded right suprarenal mass
   b. Central fluid density suggestive of necrosis.
2. I-123 MIBG SPECT scan:
   a. Increased focal uptake in the right suprarenal region
   b. No focal uptake elsewhere.

INTERPRETATION

Large I-123 MIBG-avid necrotic right adrenal mass.

MAIN DIAGNOSIS

Right adrenal phaeochromocytoma with no metastases or ectopic disease.

DIFFERENTIAL DIAGNOSIS

Right adrenal carcinoma, but this is unlikely as the tumour is MIBG positive.

FURTHER INVESTIGATIONS AND MANAGEMENT

1. Percutaneous biopsy is not recommended, especially with inadequate blood pressure control, as severe haemorrhage can result.
2. Serum and urine catecholamines and urine metanephrines.
3. Medical referral for blood pressure control and surgical referral for resection.

FURTHER INFORMATION

Phaeochromocytoma is a neuroendocrine tumour that arises from sympathetic paraganglionic tissue. Around 10% of phaeochromocytomas are extra-adrenal, 10% are bilateral, 10% are malignant and 10% are familial. Solitary lesions favour the right side. The organ of Zuckerkandl, which is near the aortic bifurcation, is the most common extra-adrenal site. Paragangliomas arising from parasympathetic cells are the glomus and carotid body tumours. MIBG scan has high sensitivity and specificity for functioning adrenal and extra-adrenal phaeochromocytomas. MIBG scan can prove especially helpful when a mass is discovered on CT, but the biochemical findings have been indeterminate.

CASE 3.3

Age: 54 years	Gender: Female
Clinical problem: Bilateral swelling of parotid glands	
Images in exam case: US (2), MRI (4)	

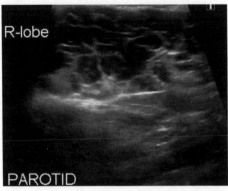

Figure 15a

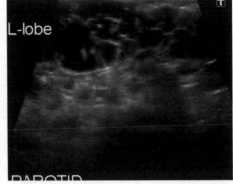

Figure 15b

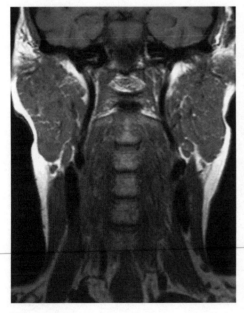

Figure 15c

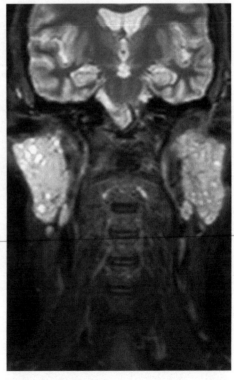

Figure 15d

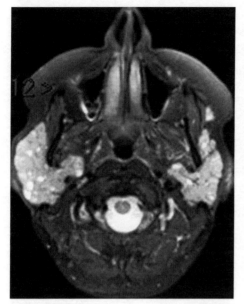

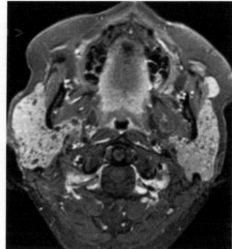

Figure 15f

Figure 15e

FINDINGS

1. Parotid ultrasonography:
   a. Multiple bilateral small cystic spaces throughout both parotid glands.
2. T1-weighted coronal MRI:
   a. Diffuse enlargement of both parotid glands
   b. Multiple low-signal foci within both parotid glands.
3. STIR coronal and axial MRI:
   a. Multiple high-signal foci within both parotid glands
   b. No focal solid mass within either parotid gland
   c. Prominent bilateral cervical lymph nodes.
4. T1-weighted fat-suppressed post-Gd axial MRI:
   a. Bilateral normal enhancement of the parotid glands with absence of enhancement of the low-signal foci.

INTERPRETATION

Bilateral diffuse enlargement of parotid glands with multiple small cystic spaces.

MAIN DIAGNOSIS

Sjögren's syndrome.

DIFFERENTIAL DIAGNOSIS

AIDS-associated lymphoepithelial lesions. This condition can be difficult to distinguish from Sjögren's syndrome, as the cross-sectional imaging appearances are almost identical. A history of HIV will help to distinguish this condition from Sjögren's syndrome.

FURTHER INVESTIGATIONS AND MANAGEMENT

1. Explore history of dry mouth and dry eyes.
2. HIV screen to rule out AIDS-associated lymphoepithelial lesions.
3. As patients with Sjögren's syndrome are at high risk of developing lymphoma, consider biopsy if a dominant intraparotid mass is identified.

FURTHER INFORMATION

Sjögren's syndrome is an autoimmune disease of the exocrine glands that causes dry eyes and xerostomia. The female:male ratio is 9:1. Sjögren's syndrome can occur either alone (primary Sjögren's) or in association with other connective tissue diseases, such as rheumatoid arthritis, systemic lupus erythematosus, scleroderma, primary biliary cirrhosis and chronic active hepatitis (secondary Sjögren's). Lymphoma is a complication of Sjögren's syndrome, and the salivary glands are the most common site of involvement. Sialography shows punctuate, globular or cavitary sialectasis. There may also be lymphoepithelial cysts and nodules. As the disease progresses, there is progressive replacement of the glandular tissue with fat.

CASE 3.4

Age: 55 years	Gender: Female
Clinical problem: Ex-smoker with shortness of breath	
Images in exam case: Plain radiograph (2), CT (4)	

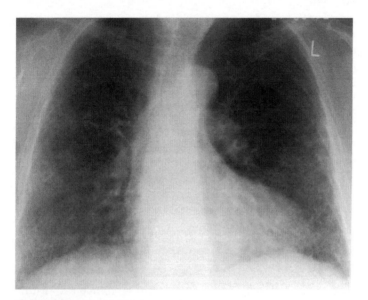

Figure 16a

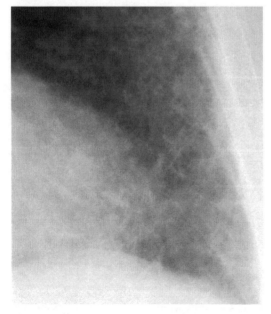

Figure 16b

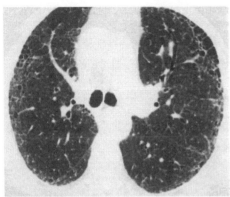

Figure 16c

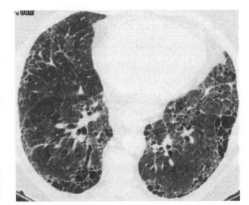
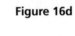

Figure 16d

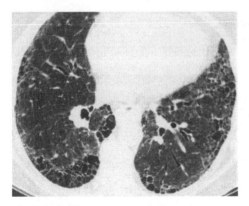

Figure 16e

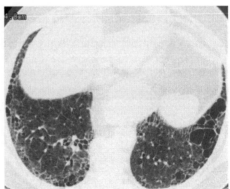

Figure 16f

FINDINGS

1. Chest X-ray:
   a. Bilateral basal predominant peripheral reticular opacification
   b. Ill-defined heart borders
   c. Normal heart size and pulmonary vascularity
   d. No calcified pleural plaques.
2. HRCT thorax:
   a. Pulmonary fibrosis as evidenced by traction bronchiectasis and bronchiolectasis
   b. Intralobular interstitial and interlobular septal thickening
   c. Subpleural honeycombing
   d. Minimal ground-glass opacification, mainly in subpleural location.

DIAGNOSIS

Interstitial pulmonary fibrosis of UIP pattern, causes of which may include:

1. Idiopathic pulmonary fibrosis
2. Asbestosis, but there are no visible pleural plaques
3. Connective tissue disease (e.g. rheumatoid arthritis, scleroderma), but there are no glenohumeral/ACJ erosions or dilated oesophagus
4. Drug-induced pulmonary fibrosis (e.g. due to bleomycin). A history of use of the offending drug would be present.

FURTHER INVESTIGATIONS AND MANAGEMENT

1. Review of previous chest X-ray or HRCT, which may show temporal heterogeneity to support the diagnosis of UIP.
2. Respiratory review with a view to identifying the potential aetiology and/or lung biopsy.

FURTHER INFORMATION

Idiopathic pulmonary fibrosis (IPF) is chronic fibrotic interstitial pneumonia of UIP pattern. UIP is characterised by heterogeneous interstitial inflammation, fibrosis and honeycombing, together with areas of normal lung. Temporal heterogeneity (i.e. the presence of acute lung injury against a background of established fibrosis) is a histological characteristic feature of UIP. The latter is a histological diagnosis, and causes include dusts (e.g. asbestos), drugs (e.g. bleomycin), collagen vascular disease (e.g. scleroderma) and hypersensitivity pneumonitis. IPF is diagnosed only after these potential causes have been excluded.

On HRCT, there is evidence of fibrosis characterised by intralobular interstitial thickening, traction bronchiolectasis and bronchiectasis, and honeycombing involving the basal and subpleural lung. There is also mild ground-glass opacification which is usually due to intralobular interstitial thickening and/or honeycombing filled with secretions. Ground-glass opacity is considered to be consistent with active inflammation only when there is no evidence of established fibrosis. The strongest predictor of IPF on HRCT is peripheral and basal honeycombing.

HRCT features that help to distinguish NSIP from UIP are as follows:

1. predominant ground-glass change that is mainly peripheral and basal
2. fibrosis and honeycombing that are generally mild
3. relative subpleural sparing
4. relative temporal and geographical homogeneity of findings.

Causes of lower zone pulmonary fibrosis (which can be remembered using the acronym CRABS) are as follows:
1. Cryptogenic fibrosing alveolitis or IPF
2. Rheumatoid arthritis
3. Asbestosis
4. Bleomycin
5. Scleroderma.

CASE 3.5

Age: 75 years	Gender: Male
Clinical problem: Back pain	
Images in exam case: Plain radiograph (1), CT (3), MRI (3)	

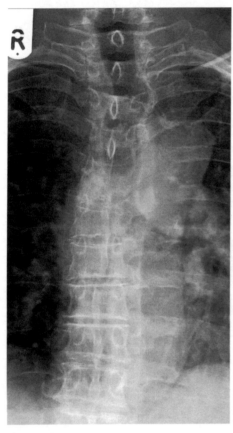

Figure 17a

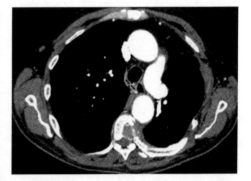

Figure 17b

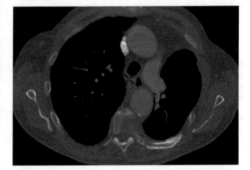

Figure 17c

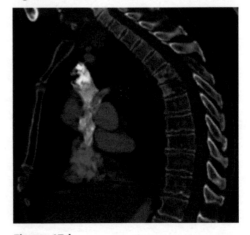

Figure 17d

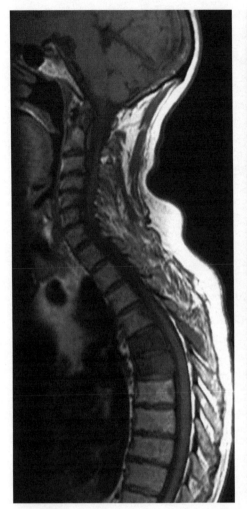

Figure 17e

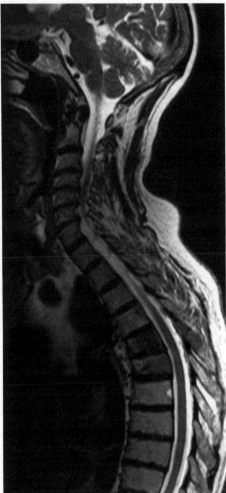

Figure 17f

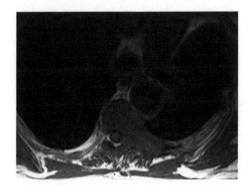

Figure 17g

FINDINGS

1. X-ray thoracic spine AP:
   a. Non-visualisation of D5 and D6 spinous processes and left pedicles.
2. CT thorax:
   a. Volume loss in the left lung, probably from previous left upper lobectomy
   b. Destruction of the left side of thoracic vertebra and left rib
   c. Large soft tissue component associated with bone destruction
   d. Soft tissue probably encroaches on the spinal canal.
3. MRI cervicothoracic spine:
   a. T1 sagittal: low-signal vertebral body D5 and D6, and a small low signal posteriorly within D4. Disc spaces are preserved
   b. T1 axial: large soft tissue mass encroaches on the spinal canal, but there is no compression of the thecal sac
   c. T2 sagittal: spinal canal is patent, and there is no spinal cord signal change.

INTERPRETATION

Multiple vertebral destructive lesions against a background of previous left upper lobectomy.

MAIN DIAGNOSIS

Multiple vertebral metastases, most probably metastatic bronchogenic carcinoma.

DIFFERENTIAL DIAGNOSIS

Multiple myeloma. However, this is less likely as the lesions are centred at the pedicles and posterior elements rather than the vertebral bodies.

FURTHER INVESTIGATIONS AND MANAGEMENT

1. Urgent oncology referral with a view to radiotherapy, as there is risk of cord compression.
2. CT-guided percutaneous biopsy of left paravertebral soft tissue.

FURTHER INFORMATION

Metastases replace the normal T1 high signal of fatty bone marrow with the low signal of tumour cells. On T2/STIR sequences, due to the higher water content, lytic metastases appear higher signal than the normal marrow. Sclerotic metastases are generally low on both T1- and T2-weighted images. Breast, prostate, lung and renal cancers are the cancers that most commonly cause spinal metastases. Foci of red marrow also appear low signal on T1 and higher signal than yellow marrow on STIR. However, normal red marrow is higher in signal than normal intervertebral discs on T1, whereas metastases are equal or lower in signal.

Generally, metastases and myeloma have identical appearances on MRI. Sometimes focal myeloma/plasmacytoma can have a 'mini-brain' appearance, which helps to distinguish it from metastasis. A separate variegated pattern can also be seen with myeloma, in which marrow appears as if black pepper has been sprinkled over fatty marrow on T1 images. In addition, myeloma can have large soft tissue components.

CASE 3.6

Age: 75 years	Gender: Male
Clinical problem: History of prostate cancer, and recent development of back pain	
Images in exam case: Bone scan (1), MRI (5)	

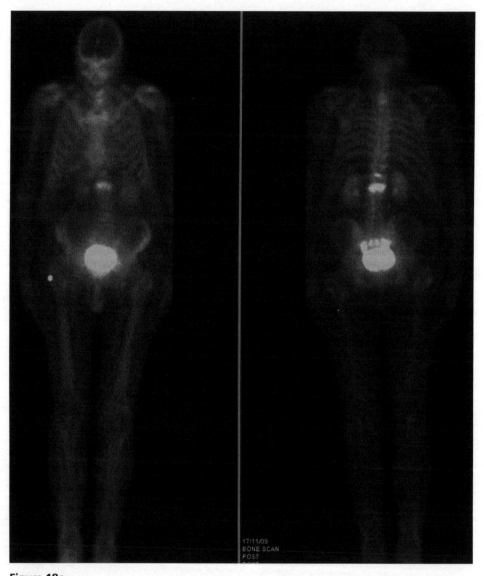

17/11/09
BONE SCAN
POST

Figure 18a

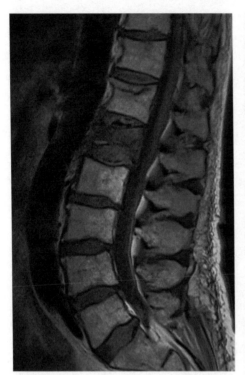

Figure 18b

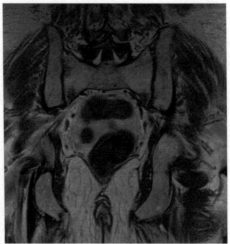

Figure 18c

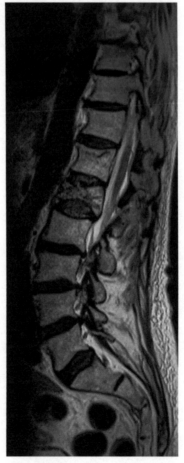

Figure 18d

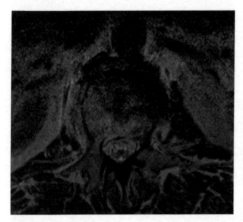

Figure 18e

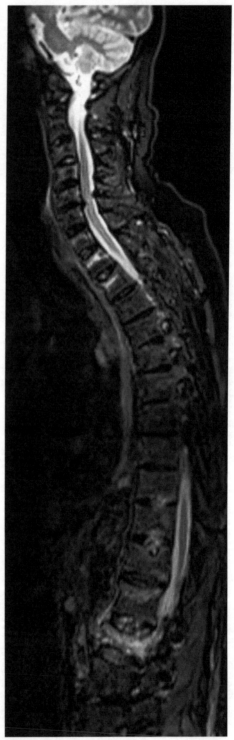

Figure 18f

FINDINGS

1. Bone scan:
   a. Increased uptake in D12 and L1 vertebral bodies and within the sacrum
   b. Slightly increased uptake also seen in D1 and D2 vertebral bodies.
2. MRI:
   a. T1 sagittal lumbar spine: low-signal fracture line through the mid L1 vertebral body associated with low-signal marrow throughout the vertebral body. Low-signal sub-endplate fracture line D12 with mild marrow signal change on either side of the fracture line
   b. T1 coronal sacrum: low-signal fracture lines across both sacral alae
   c. T2 sagittal lumbar spine: compression fracture L1 and superior sub-endplate fracture D12. Bulging of L1 vertebral body into the spinal canal, but no significant spinal canal stenosis
   d. T2 axial at L1: no significant paraspinal mass, and no posterior element involvement
   e. STIR sagittal whole spine: STIR high signal D12 and superior aspect L1 vertebral body. High signal also in the superior aspects of D1 and D2, consistent with further endplate compression fractures.

INTERPRETATION

Acute fractures of D1, D2, D12 and L1 vertebral bodies and both sacral alae as evidenced by T1 low signal and STIR high signal consistent with marrow oedema.

MAIN DIAGNOSIS

Insufficiency fractures.

DIFFERENTIAL DIAGNOSIS

1. Pathological fractures secondary to metastases. However, this is less likely as the posterior elements are not involved, marrow signal change is patchy and the fracture sites are typical of insufficiency fractures.
2. Old healed compression fractures. However, this is less likely as these have normal marrow signal on all sequences.

FURTHER INVESTIGATIONS AND MANAGEMENT

1. Medical referral for pain relief, rest and rehabilitation, and risk factor reduction programme.
2. Interventional radiology referral for consideration of vertebroplasty.

FURTHER INFORMATION

Insufficiency fractures result from normal stress applied to abnormal bone. The typical sites are vertebral bodies, sacrum, supra-acetabular region, pubic rami and femoral neck.

The most common cause is osteoporosis, but these fractures can also occur with steroid therapy, Paget's disease, osteomalacia and post irradiation.

On MRI, the typical appearance of an acute insufficiency fracture is a T1 low-signal fracture line associated with low T1 and high T2/STIR signal oedema. Distinguishing insufficiency fractures from pathological fractures secondary to malignancy can be difficult, but a sharp margin between normal and abnormal marrow within the affected vertebral body, lack of posterior element involvement and the absence of paraspinal soft tissue are signs indicative of a benign aetiology.

The Honda sign in radionuclide bone scan is an 'H-shaped' uptake within the sacrum secondary to sacral insufficiency fracture.

Case bag 4

CASE 4.1

Age: 24 years	Gender: Male
Clinical problem: Epilepsy	
Images in exam case: MRI (8)	

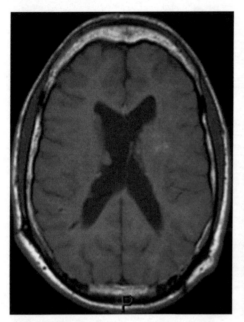

Figure 19a

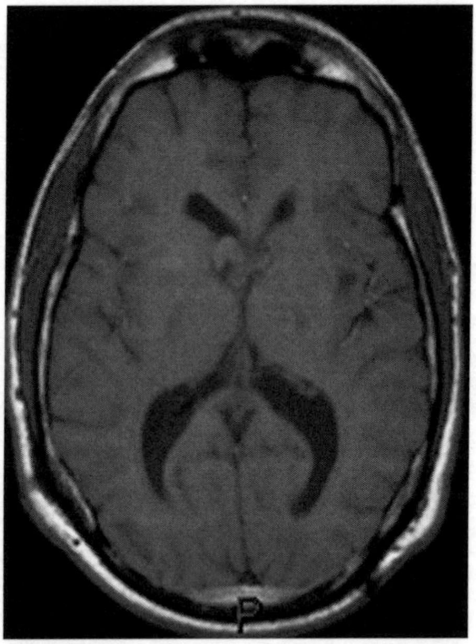

Figure 19b

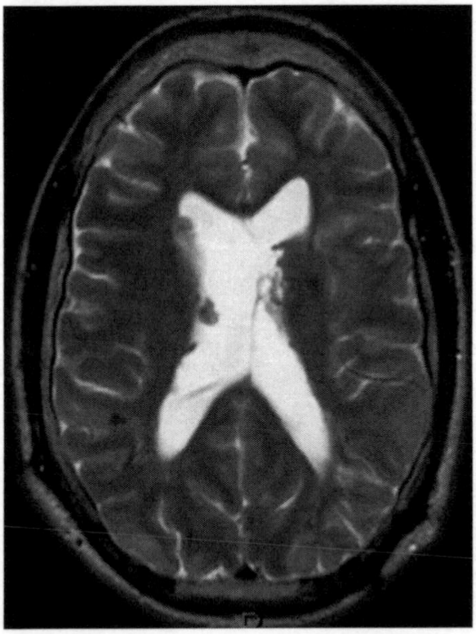

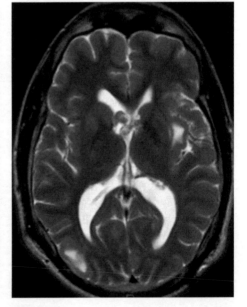

Figure 19c

Figure 19d

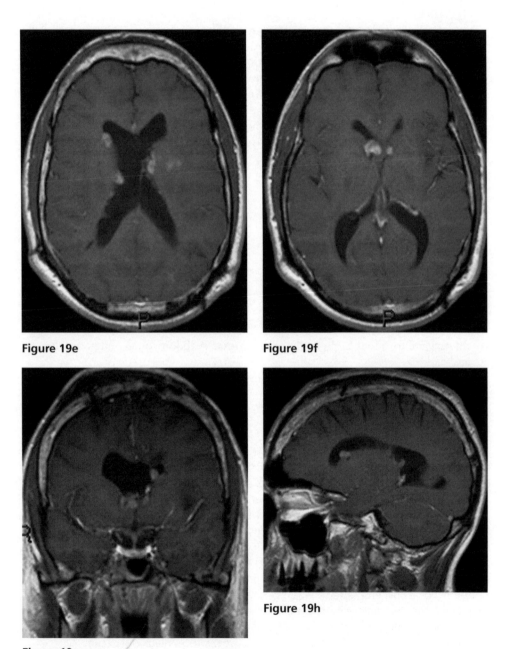

Figure 19e

Figure 19f

Figure 19g

Figure 19h

FINDINGS

1. Pre-contrast T1 axial:
    a. Multiple isointense subependymal nodules along both lateral ventricles
    b. Small lobulated mass at the foramen of Monro
    c. Cortical thickening and low signal at the right occipital lobe and left insular cortex.
2. T2 axial:
    a. Subependymal nodules are isointense to the grey matter
    b. The mass at the foramen of Monro is isointense to minimally hyperintense
    c. Cortical thickening associated with high signal extends subcortically at the right occipital lobe and left insular cortex.
3. Post-contrast T1 axial, sagittal and coronal:
    a. Homogeneous enhancement of the subependymal nodules
    b. Heterogeneous enhancement of the mass at the foramen of Monro
    c. No enhancement of the right occipital and left insular cortex lesions
    d. CSF shunt/access device *in situ* on the right.

INTERPRETATION

Subependymal nodules, cortical tubers and probable giant-cell astrocytoma at the foramen of Monro.

DIAGNOSIS

Tuberous sclerosis.

FURTHER INVESTIGATIONS AND MANAGEMENT

1. Investigate for renal angiomyolipomas, cardiac rhabdomyomas and pulmonary cystic disease.
2. Neurology review for medical management of epilepsy.
3. Screening of family members.

FURTHER INFORMATION

Tuberous sclerosis, also known as Bourneville disease, can be familial (autosomal dominant, chromosome 9 or 16) or spontaneous. CNS features include cortical tubers, subependymal nodules, white matter hamartomas and subependymal giant-cell astrocytomas. Extra-CNS features include adenoma sebaceum, shagreen patches and subungal fibromas (cutaneous), renal angiomyolipomas, pulmonary cystic disease, retinal hamartomas, cardiac rhabdomyomas and cystic osseous lesions. Patients present with epilepsy and mental retardation.

Cortical tubers are hypointense on T1 and hyperintense on T2, with variable enhancement. Subependymal nodules resemble 'candle drippings', are iso- to hyperintense on T1 and hypo- to hyperintense on T2, and may show some contrast enhancement. Subependymal nodules can calcify. Giant-cell astrocytoma occurs adjacent to the foramen of Monro, and is hypo- to isointense on T1 and iso- to hyperintense on T2, with moderate enhancement on post-contrast images. Obstructive hydrocephalus can occur.

CASE 4.2

Age: 60 years	Gender: Female
Clinical problem: Neck pain and upper motor neuron signs in the upper limbs	
Images in exam case: CT (2), MRI (6)	

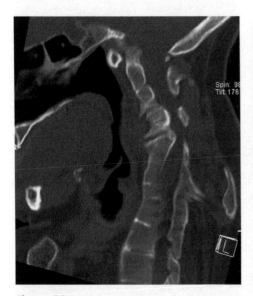

Figure 20a

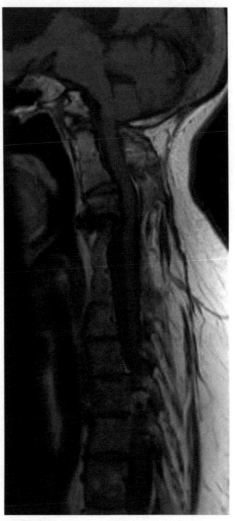

Figure 20c

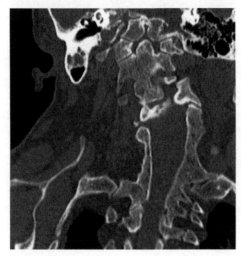

Figure 20b

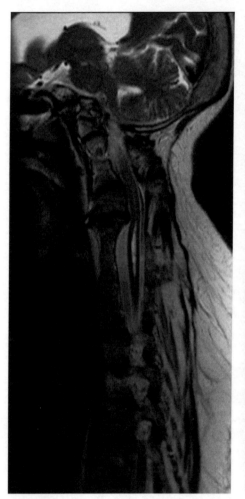

Figure 20d

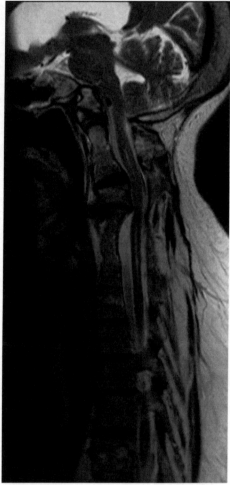

Figure 20e

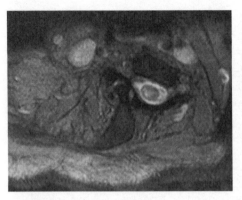

Figure 20f

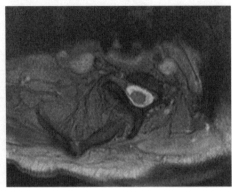

Figure 20g

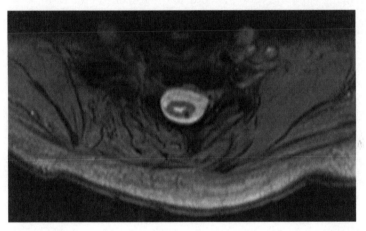

Figure 20h

FINDINGS

1. CT cervical spine:
   a. C4–7 congenital block vertebra
   b. Fusion of corresponding posterior elements
   c. Kyphoscoliosis with convexity to the left
   d. High-lying scapula (Sprengel's deformity).
2. T1 sagittal MRI:
   a. C4–7 block vertebra
   b. Patent craniocervical junction
   c. Thickened skull vault.
3. T2 sagittal and axial MRI:
   a. Syrinx within the cervical spinal cord extending from mid-C2 to C6 level
   b. Dilated ventriculo-sulcal system
   c. Bony bar extending from the vertebral body to the scapula on the right
   d. Tiny low-signal focus posteriorly within the spinal cord, most probably a cavernous malformation.

INTERPRETATION

Congenital segmentation anomaly of cervical spine with high-lying scapula, omovertebral bone and associated syringomyelia.

MAIN DIAGNOSIS

1. Klippel–Feil syndrome.
2. Tiny cavernoma of the cervical spinal cord.

DIFFERENTIAL DIAGNOSIS

1. Ankylosing spondylitis. However, there is no evidence of ossification of longitudinal ligaments.
2. Rheumatoid arthritis. However, there are no erosions, there is no angulation at the vertebral fusion site and the spinous processes are also fused, which are features against this diagnosis.

FURTHER INVESTIGATIONS AND MANAGEMENT

1. Search for other associated congenital anomalies if these have not already been ascertained (e.g. renal, auditory and cardiovascular anomalies).
2. Flexion–extension views may be necessary to look for a hypermobile/unstable segment.
3. Orthopaedic/neurosurgical review.

FURTHER INFORMATION

Klippel–Feil syndrome is a vertebral segmentation anomaly characterised by fusion of multiple cervical vertebral bodies, including the posterior elements. The neck is short, with limited movement. Other associated anomalies are Sprengel's shoulder (high position of the scapula), scoliosis, omovertebral bone, cervical ribs, rib fusion, and deafness due to ear anomalies. There may be platybasia, syringomyelia, encephalocoele and craniofacial asymmetry. Congenital heart diseases and genitourinary abnormalities may also be present.

CASE 4.3

Age: 65 years	Gender: Male
Clinical problem: Chest pain and shortness of breath	
Images in exam case: Plain radiograph (1), CT (7)	

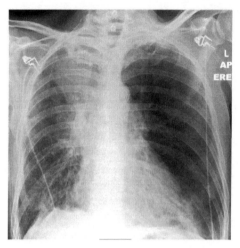

Figure 21a

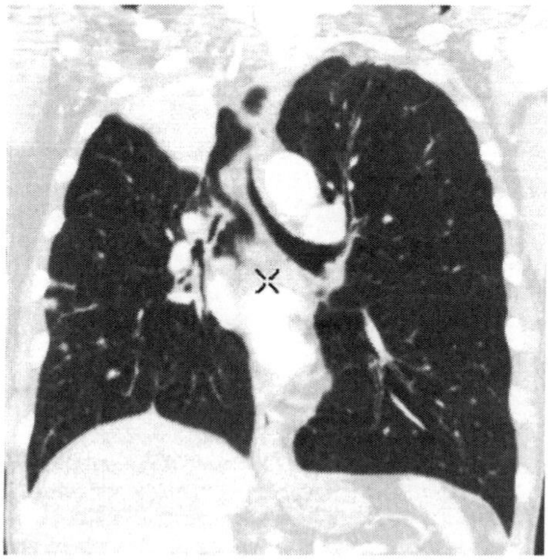

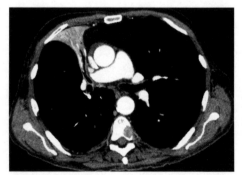

Figure 21b

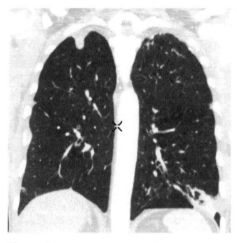

Figure 21c

Figure 21d

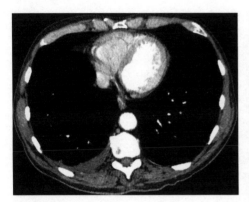

Figure 21e

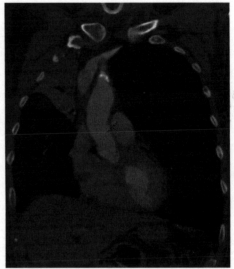

Figure 21f

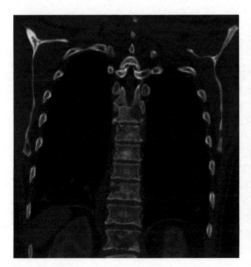

Figure 21g

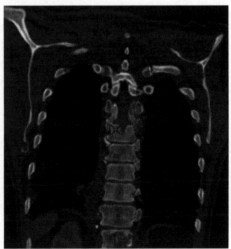

Figure 21h

FINDINGS

1. Chest X-ray:
    a. Right upper lobe opacification
    b. Volume loss of right upper lobe – elevated right hilum, upward deviation of the minor fissure and ipsilateral hilar shift
    c. Pathological posterior right 5th rib fracture
    d. Left basal consolidation.
2. CT thorax:
    a. Right upper lobe collapse
    b. Pulmonary nodules in the right lower lobe
    c. Lytic lesions in the vertebral bodies and left scapula
    d. Centrilobular emphysema
    e. Small right pleural effusion.

DIAGNOSIS

Bronchogenic carcinoma causing right upper lobe collapse, multiple lytic bone metastases and pathological right 5th rib fracture, and multiple pulmonary metastases.

FURTHER INVESTIGATIONS AND MANAGEMENT

1. Urgent respiratory referral with a view to bronchoscopic biopsy.
2. Lung cancer MDT review.

FURTHER INFORMATION

The salient features of the new TNM (7th edition) staging of lung cancer are as follows:

*   T staging: T1a < 2 cm, T1b 2–3 cm, T2a 3–5 cm, T2b 5–7 cm and T3 > 7 cm (previously T1 and T2 had cut-off values of 3 cm). Satellite nodules in the same lobe are classified as T3 (previously T4). Tumour invading the chest wall, including superior sulcus, diaphragm, mediastinal pleura or parietal pericardium, tumour within 2 cm of carina or tumour causing distal collapse or pneumonitis, is classified as T3. Tumour invading the mediastinum, heart, great vessels, trachea, recurrent laryngeal nerve, oesophagus, vertebral body or carina is classified as T4. Metastatic nodule in a separate lobe but within ipsilateral lung is also classified as T4 (previously M1).
*   N staging: This is essentially similar, except that nodal stations are now better defined. N1 is ipsilateral peribronchial, hilar or intrapulmonary lymph nodes. N2 is ipsilateral mediastinal or subcarinal lymph nodes. N3 is contralateral hilar, contralateral mediastinal or ipsilateral or contralateral supraclavicular or scalene nodes.
*   M staging: Malignant pleural or pericardial effusion is M1a. Lung nodules in a separate lobe but ipsilateral lung are T4 (previously M1). Contralateral lung nodules are M1a. All metastases outside the lungs are M1b.

CASE 4.4

Age: 20 years	Gender: Female
Clinical problem: Sudden loss of consciousness	
Images in exam case: MRI (8)	

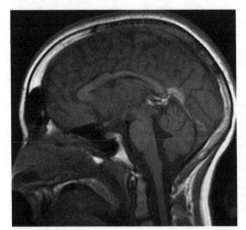

Figure 22a

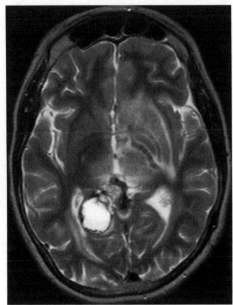

Figure 22b

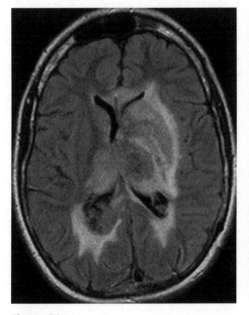

Figure 22c

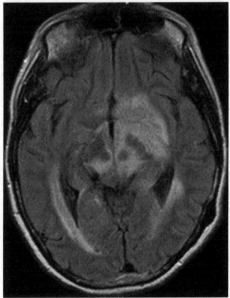

Figure 22d

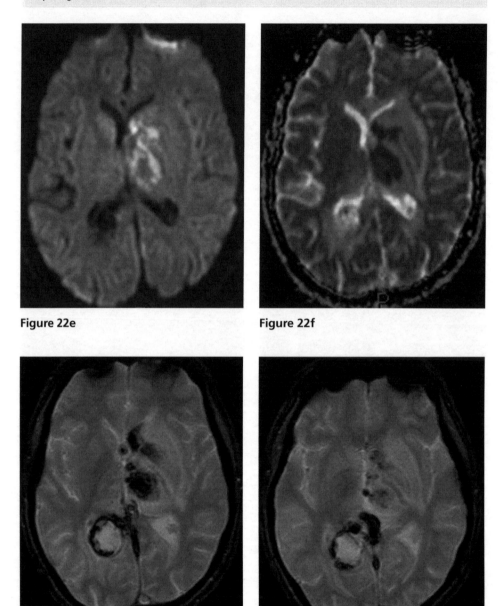

Figure 22e

Figure 22f

Figure 22g

Figure 22h

FINDINGS

1. T1 sagittal:
   a. High signal within the internal cerebral veins, vein of Galen and straight sinus.
2. FLAIR and T2 axials:
   a. High signal within the left basal ganglia, bilateral thalami and brainstem
   b. Mass effect causing partial effacement of the left lateral ventricle
   c. Rounded heterogeneous high-signal mass with low-signal rim, adjacent to the occipital horn of the right lateral ventricle.
3. DWI and ADC maps:
   a. Diffusion restriction within the left thalamus and basal ganglia
   b. No diffusion restriction within the right occipital mass.
4. GRE T2 axial:
   a. Low signal within left thalamus, basal ganglia, anterior rim of the right occipital mass and vein of Galen.

DIAGNOSIS

1. Deep cerebral venous thrombosis causing haemorrhagic infarction of the left thalamus and basal ganglia, and ischaemia of the right thalamus.
2. Cavernous malformation of the right occipital lobe.

FURTHER INVESTIGATIONS AND MANAGEMENT

1. MR venogram to assess the true extent of thrombus.
2. Neurology referral for further management of deep cerebral venous thrombosis.

FURTHER INFORMATION

MRI of blood is summarised below:
- Oxyhaemoglobin (hyperacute haemorrhage, < 6 hours): diamagnetic, low T1 and high T2
- Deoxyhaemoglobin (acute haemorrhage, 8–72 hours): paramagnetic, low T1 (susceptibility) and low T2 (susceptibility)
- Intracellular methaemoglobin (early subacute, 3–7 days): paramagnetic, high T1 (proton–dipole interaction) and low T2 (susceptibility)
- Free methaemoglobin (late subacute, 1 week to months): paramagnetic, high T1 (proton–dipole interaction) and high T2 (proton–dipole interaction)
- Haemosiderin and ferritin (chronic, months to years): superparamagnetic, low T1 and T2 (susceptibility effects).

Spin echo sequences use at least two radiofrequency pulses, namely an excitation pulse and one or more 180-degree refocusing pulses. As the proton dephasing occurs following an initial excitation pulse through T2* relaxation processes, causing them to lose transverse coherence, a refocusing pulse is applied. A refocusing pulse causes the protons to reverse their phases, allowing the protons to regain their transverse coherence, producing a signal called *spin echo*. Due to application of this refocusing pulse, the main magnetic field inhomogeneity and susceptibility differences are eliminated.

Gradient echo sequences do not use 180-degree pulses to refocus the protons, but instead use a gradient to reduce the magnetic inhomogeneity effects. A gradient changes the magnetic field strength, which in turn changes the precessional frequency and the phase of spins, causing them to rephase. Gradient rephasing is less efficient than radiofrequency rephrasing, and thus the gradient echo sequences are more sensitive to magnetic field inhomogeneities.

CASE 4.5

Age: 49 years	Gender: Female
Clinical problem: Ankle swelling	
Images in exam case: Plain radiograph (2), MRI (4)	

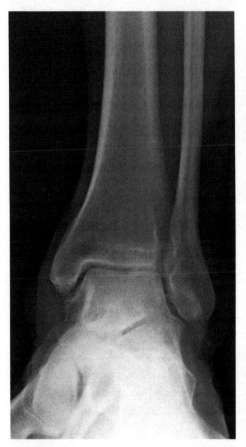

Figure 23a

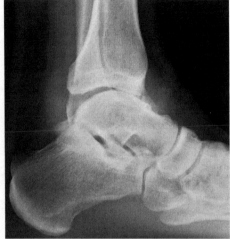

Figure 23b

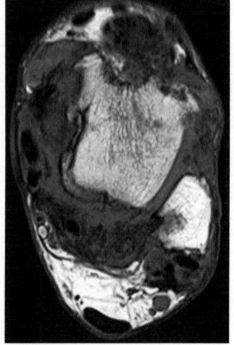

Figure 23c

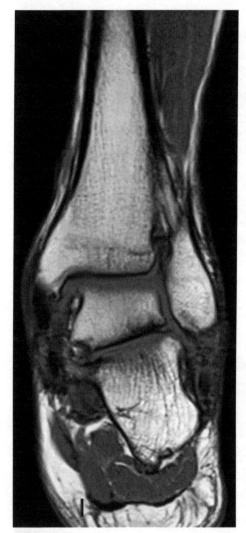

Figure 23d

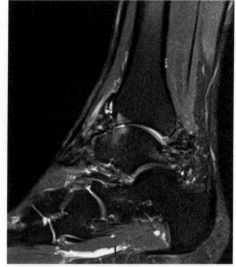

Figure 23e

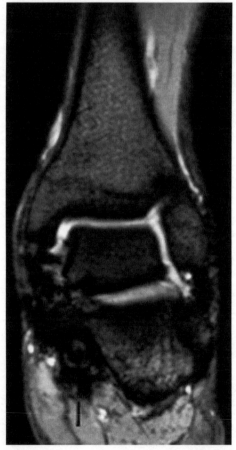

Figure 23f

FINDINGS

1. X-ray ankle: Extensive soft tissue swelling overlying ankle joint.
2. T1 coronal and axial:
   a. Low-signal soft tissue thickening around the ankle and subtalar joints
   b. Joint spaces preserved.
3. STIR sagittal: Low-signal soft tissue thickening around the ankle and subtalar joints.
4. GRE T2 coronal: Signal drop within thickened periarticular soft tissues with 'blooming' artefact in GRE T2 images.

INTERPRETATION

Low T1 signal synovial hypertrophy with blooming on gradient-echo images most probably due to haemosiderin deposition.

MAIN DIAGNOSIS

Pigmented villonodular synovitis of left ankle joint.

DIFFERENTIAL DIAGNOSIS

1. Gout. However, there are no erosions. There would also be a long history of joint pain, particularly affecting the first metatarsophalangeal joints.
2. Amyloid deposition. This usually occurs in patients with severe chronic kidney disease on haemodialysis.
3. Non-calcified synovial osteochondromatosis. However, there are no cartilaginous deposits and/or loose bodies within the joint.

FURTHER INFORMATION

Pigmented villonodular synovitis (PVNS) is due to chronic benign proliferation of synovium. There is joint swelling secondary to synovial thickening and effusion. Haemosiderin deposition is due to repeated haemorrhage. Giant-cell tumour of tendon sheath represents the same pathology affecting the tendon sheath instead of a joint or bursa. The thickened synovium almost never calcifies. Cystic erosions and joint space narrowing are late features of PVNS.

CASE 4.6

Age: 38 years	Gender: Female
Clinical problem: Back pain	
Images in exam case: Plain radiograph (2), MRI (4)	

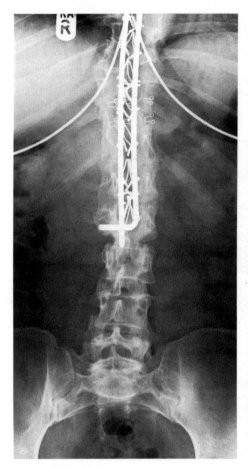

Figure 24a

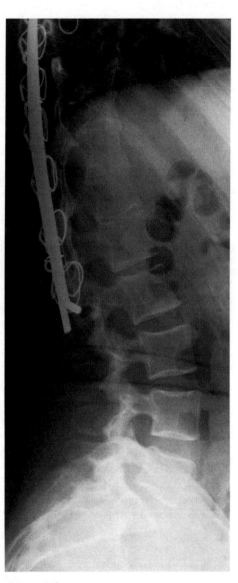

Figure 24b

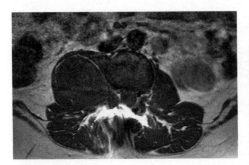

Figure 24c

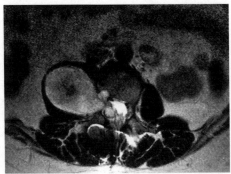

Figure 24e

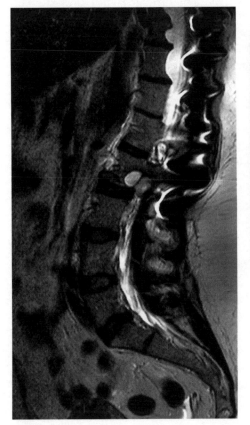

Figure 24d

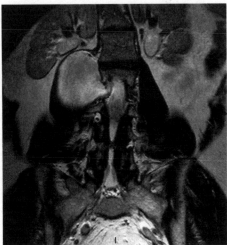

Figure 24f

FINDINGS

1. X-ray lumbar spine:
   a. Thoracolumbar spinal fixation with a pair of rods and wires
   b. Posterior scalloping of lower thoracic vertebral bodies (D10/11).
2. T1 axial:
   a. Low-signal well-defined paraspinal mass extending through the neural foramen into the spinal canal
   b. Thinning and displacement of the right psoas muscle. Fat plane between the muscle and tumour is preserved
   c. Metallic artefacts.
3. T2 sagittal, coronal and axial:
   a. Dumb-bell-shaped high-signal mass extending through right L2 neural foramen into the spinal canal
   b. Central low signal within the mass
   c. Widened L2 neural foramen
   d. Posterior scalloping of lower thoracic vertebrae (D10/11)
   e. Metallic artefacts.

INTERPRETATION

Large right L2 neurofibroma with dural ectasia giving rise to posterior scalloping of thoracic vertebrae. Previous corrective rod fixation for scoliosis.

DIAGNOSIS

Neurofibromatosis type 1 (NF-1).

FURTHER INVESTIGATIONS AND MANAGEMENT

Neurosurgical referral.

FURTHER INFORMATION

NF-1 is sporadic in 50% and hereditary in 50% of cases. The hereditary form is autosomal dominant with a defective chromosome 17. Patients may develop optic pathway gliomas (pilocytic astrocytomas), and cerebellar, brainstem and cerebral astrocytomas. On MRI T2 bright signal foci may be seen on the brainstem, basal ganglia and cerebellum (neurofibromatosis bright objects, NBOs). Multiple peripheral neurofibromas, large plexiform neurofibromas, spinal dural ectasia, posterior vertebral scalloping, aqueductal stenosis, lateral thoracic meningocoeles, sphenoid wing hypoplasia, bowing of tibia and fibula, pseudoarthrosis, ribbon ribs, renal artery stenosis, coarctation of abdominal aorta and phaeochromocytoma are all features of NF-1.

Case bag 5

CASE 5.1

Age: 42 years	Gender: Female
Clinical problem: Right upper quadrant pain	
Images in exam case: MRI (9)	

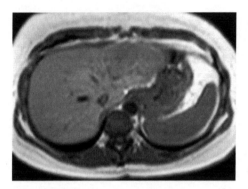

Figure 25a

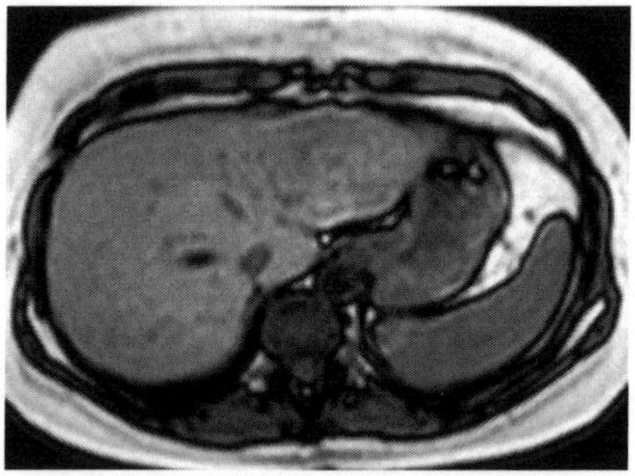

Figure 25b

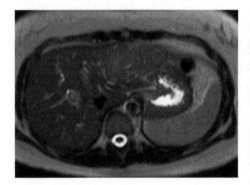

Figure 25c

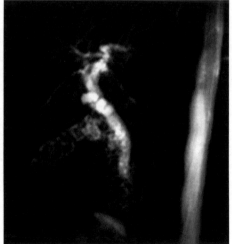

Figure 25d

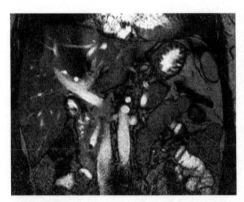

Figure 25e

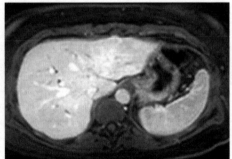

Figure 25f

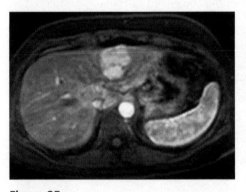

Figure 25g

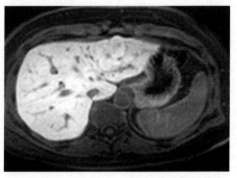

Figure 25h

Figure 25i

FINDINGS

1. Pre-contrast T1-weighted images:
   a. Isointense, well-defined mass within the left lobe of liver
   b. Central hypointense scar within the mass
   c. No loss of signal in opposed phase image.
2. T2-weighted images:
   a. The lesion is minimally hyperintense
   b. The gallbladder is packed with stones in cholangiographic sequences
   c. Intra- and extrahepatic bile ducts are dilated
   d. Distal common bile duct has a filling defect, consistent with a calculus.
3. Post-contrast T1-weighted images:
   a. Left liver mass enhances on arterial phase
   b. Central scar does not enhance on arterial phase
   c. The lesion is isointense to liver parenchyma on venous phase
   d. On delayed hepatobiliary phase, the lesion is iso- to minimally hyperintense relative to liver parenchyma.

MAIN DIAGNOSIS

1. Focal nodular hyperplasia (FNH) of the left lobe of liver.
2. Cholelithiasis and choledocholithiasis causing intra- and extrahepatic biliary dilatation.

DIFFERENTIAL DIAGNOSIS

1. Hepatic adenoma. However, this is less likely as the lesion does not contain fat or a pseudocapsule. In addition, adenomas are less likely to have a central scar than FNH.
2. Fibrolamellar hepatocellular carcinoma. However, this is less likely as the scar in FNH is generally low signal on both T1 and T2, enhancement is heterogeneous in both the arterial and portovenous phase, and the central scar does not usually enhance.

FURTHER INVESTIGATIONS AND MANAGEMENT

1. Surgical referral for ERCP and cholecystectomy.
2. Increasing pain and progressive disease may necessitate surgery for the FNH – referral to hepatobiliary team.

FURTHER INFORMATION

Focal nodular hyperplasia is a rare benign tumour that is most common in young females. It has been proposed that FNH is a hyperplastic hepatic parenchymal response to an arterial malformation. The central scar contains malformed blood vessels. FNH has no malignant potential. It is generally a solitary lesion. However, multiple FNH syndrome also exists, and is associated with hepatic haemangioma, meningioma, astrocytoma, berry aneurysm and portal vein atresia. On post-contrast images, the arterial phase enhancement is intense and uniform, rapidly becoming isointense to the parenchyma. FNH contains functioning hepatocytes but no functional portal tracts or connecting biliary drainage, hence it is hyperintense to liver parenchyma in delayed images.

Hepatic adenoma is associated with oral contraceptive steroid use, galactosaemia and glycogen storage disease. Hepatic adenoma can contain microscopic fat, resulting in signal loss in out-of-phase MRI. Fibrolamellar hepatocellular carcinoma occurs in young patients, generally females, without background chronic liver disease. Serum alpha fetoprotein is usually normal. The central scar is irregular, is generally larger than that found in FNH, and is hypointense on both T1- and T2-weighted images. On post-contrast images the enhancement is intense but heterogeneous, and may persist in the portovenous phase. The scar in FNH is generally small, whereas the scar in fibrolamellar HCC is large, and enhancement is heterogeneous and negligible.

CASE 5.2

Age: 48 years	Gender: Male
Clinical problem: Haemoptysis	
Images in exam case: Plain radiograph (1), CT (5)	

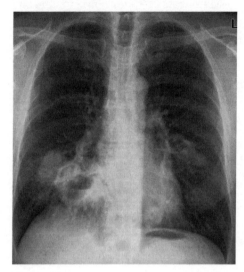

Figure 26a

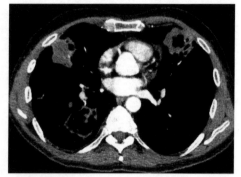

Figure 26b

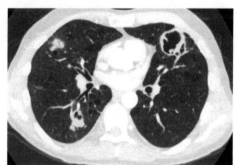

Figure 26c

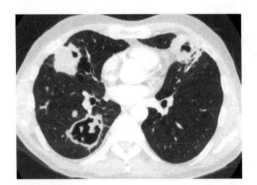

Figure 26d

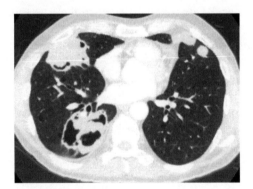

Figure 26e

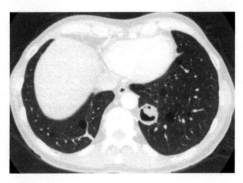

Figure 26f

FINDINGS

1. Chest X-ray:
   a. Multiple soft tissue masses in left mid and lower zones and right lower zones
   b. Some of the masses are cavitating
   c. Air-fluid level in right lower lobe mass.
2. CT thorax:
   a. Multiple bilateral thick-walled cavitating lung lesions in lingula, right middle and right lower lobes. Cavities have an irregular inner margin
   b. Solid non-cavitating lesion in the left lingula
   c. Background emphysema
   d. No lymph node enlargement.

INTERPRETATION

Multiple bilateral cavitary and non-cavitary lung masses.

DIFFERENTIAL DIAGNOSIS

Use the acronym CAVIT:
1. **C**ancer: metastatic squamous-cell carcinoma
2. **A**utoimmune: Wegener's granulomatosis, necrobiotic rheumatoid nodules
3. **V**ascular: pulmonary infarction
4. **I**nfection: staphylococcal, tuberculous, klebsiella
5. **T**rauma: cavitating haematoma, pulmonary laceration.

FURTHER INVESTIGATIONS AND MANAGEMENT

1. Review of previous imaging.
2. Respiratory referral.
3. CT-guided biopsy.

FURTHER INFORMATION

Multiple cavitating lung lesions have a wide differential diagnosis. The acronym CAVIT is a quick memory aid. The above case is that of Wegener's granulomatosis, which is a form of granulomatous vasculitis of small to medium-sized vessels. The respiratory tract and kidneys (glomerulonephritis) are affected. Patients present with sinusitis, haemoptysis, haematuria, proteinuria and renal failure. C-ANCA is positive in up to 90% of patients with active disease. Radiographic findings are solitary or multiple masses which are often cavitary, and focal or diffuse consolidation, usually secondary to pulmonary haemorrhage. Pleural effusion/thickening and lymph node enlargement can also occur.

CASE 5.3

Age: 22 years	Gender: Female
Clinical problem: Amenorrhoea	
Images in exam case: MRI (2)	

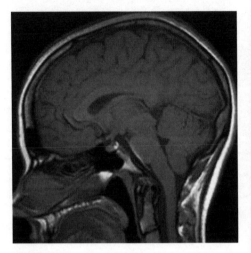

Figure 27a

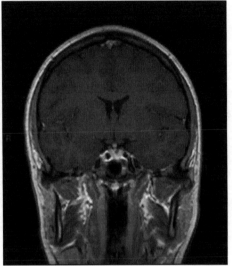

Figure 27b

FINDINGS

1. Pre-contrast T1 sagittal:
   a. Normal pituitary stalk and pituitary gland
   b. Sella not enlarged
   c. Normal appearance of the rest of the brain.
2. Post-contrast T1 coronal:
   a. Tiny focus of low signal to the left of midline within the pituitary gland
   b. The rest of the pituitary gland appears to enhance homogeneously with no glandular enlargement
   c. Normal optic chiasm and cavernous sinuses.

DIAGNOSIS

Pituitary microadenoma.

DIFFERENTIAL DIAGNOSIS

Rathke's cleft cyst.

FURTHER INVESTIGATIONS AND MANAGEMENT

1. Pituitary hormone assay.
2. Neuroendocrine referral.

FURTHER INFORMATION

Differential enhancement of the pituitary gland relative to pituitary microadenoma (<10 mm) aids detection of microadenomas on dynamic contrast-enhanced MRI or CT. The greatest contrast between normally enhancing gland and hypo-enhancing adenoma is best observed in the first minute post-contrast images. In delayed scan, microadenoma may be hyperintense relative to the rest of the gland. Contrast also helps to assess cavernous sinus invasion, with lack of immediate enhancement indicating invasion. ACTH-secreting pituitary adenomas are the smallest of all pituitary adenomas.

CASE 5.4

Age: 43 years	Gender: Female
Clinical problem: History of one week of neck pain and one day of right arm weakness	
Images in exam case: MRI (5)	

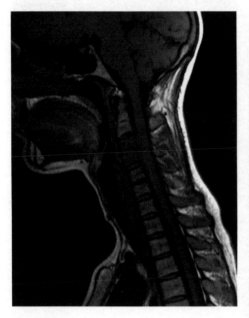

Figure 28a

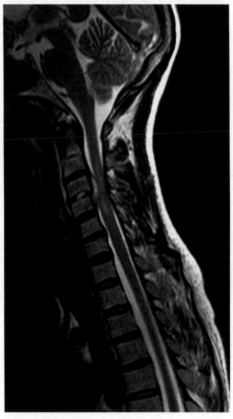

Figure 28b

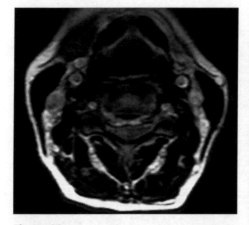

Figure 28c

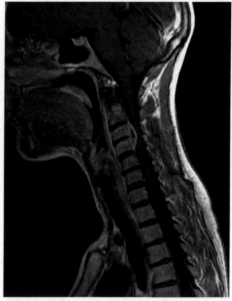

Figure 28d

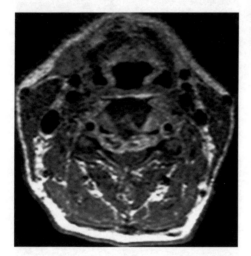

Figure 28e

FINDINGS

1. T1 pre-Gd sagittal:
   a. Low-signal bone marrow of C3 and C4 vertebral bodies
   b. Low-signal epidural thickening posterior to C3 and C4.
2. T2 sagittal:
   a. High-signal epidural collection posterior to C3 and C4
   b. Spinal cord compression by the epidural collection with T2 high-signal change within the cord
   c. High signal within C3/4 intervertebral disc but no adjacent endplate destruction.
3. T1 post-Gd:
   a. Peripheral enhancement of the epidural collection
   b. No enhancement of the C3/4 intervertebral disc.

MAIN DIAGNOSIS

C3/4 discitis with spinal epidural abscess causing spinal cord compression.

DIFFERENTIAL DIAGNOSIS

1. Tuberculosis. However, generally there is relative sparing of the disc space, the paraspinal component is large, and multiple levels can be affected as infection spreads underneath the anterior spinal ligament. The history is rather prolonged and there is often bone destruction and spinal deformity by the time of diagnosis.
2. Metastasis. However, disc space is rarely affected by metastasis, and enhancement is usually solid rather than peripheral.

FURTHER INVESTIGATIONS AND MANAGEMENT

1. Urgent neurosurgical referral for decompression.
2. Culture of fluid/tissue obtained at surgery.

FURTHER INFORMATION

Staphylococcus aureus is the organism that most commonly causes epidural abscess. Infection first affects the vertebral endplates and spreads to the intervertebral disc and then directly into the epidural space. Epidural infection may sometimes occur directly from haematogenous spread, or rarely from secondary infection of an epidural haematoma.

Tubercular infection of the spine can be clinically indolent. By the time of diagnosis, there is generally evidence of bone destruction and deformity. The disc spaces are relatively spared until late in the disease process. Infection spreads beneath the anterior or posterior longitudinal ligaments and multiple levels can become affected. The paraspinal collections are common and large at the time of diagnosis.

CASE 5.5

Age: 38 years	Gender: Female
Clinical problem: A history of five weeks of headache	
Images in exam case: CT (1), MRI (5)	

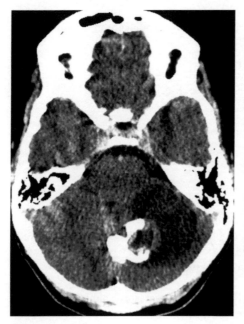

Figure 29a

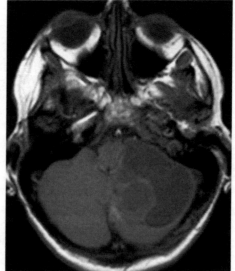

Figure 29b

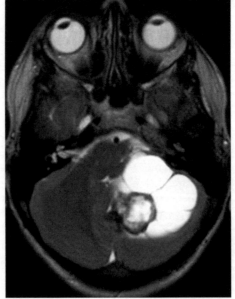

Figure 29c

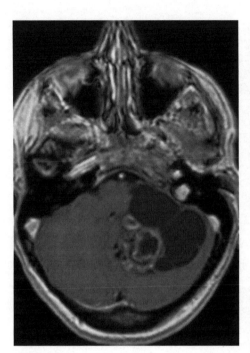

Figure 29d

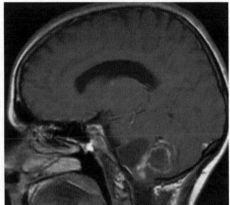

Figure 29e

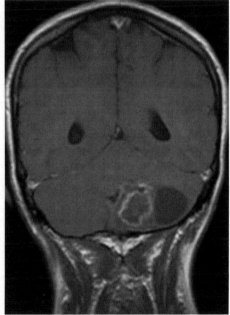

Figure 29f

FINDINGS

1. CT brain:
    a. Mixed solid and cystic mass arising from the left cerebellar hemisphere and extending into the left cerebellopontine angle cistern
    b. Coarse calcifications at the medial aspect of the mass
    c. Mass effect with mild midline shift to the right.
2. MRI brain:
    a. Large heterogeneous mass arising from the left cerebellar hemisphere
    b. The mass is predominantly low signal on T1 and high signal on T2, with intermediate signal in the medial aspect of the mass
    c. Mass effect compressing and displacing the brainstem to the right and partially effacing the fourth ventricle. There is no hydrocephalus
    d. Minimal surrounding oedema
    e. Heterogeneous ring enhancement of the medial aspect of the mass.

INTERPRETATION

Partly calcified mixed solid and cystic left cerebellar mass with peripheral enhancement of the solid components.

MAIN DIAGNOSIS

Pilocytic astrocytoma of the left cerebellum causing mass effect that is compressing and displacing the brainstem.

DIFFERENTIAL DIAGNOSIS

1. Haemangioblastoma. The solid component is usually highly vascular with avid enhancement. The mural nodule is usually tiny in comparison with a large cystic component. Calcification does not occur. Haemangioblastomas can be associated with von Hippel–Lindau syndrome.
2. Ganglioglioma. However, the commonest site of this tumour is the temporal lobe.

FURTHER INVESTIGATIONS AND MANAGEMENT

Urgent neurosurgical referral.

FURTHER INFORMATION

Pilocytic astrocytoma is the commonest posterior fossa tumour among the paediatric age group. This case is unusual, as the patient is in her late thirties. This is a benign subtype (WHO grade I) of astrocytoma, and is generally a cystic mass with a mural nodule arising from the cyst wall. Cerebellar haemangioblastoma is also a benign tumour, and is the commonest primary posterior fossa tumour in adults. However, the presence of calcifications in this case argues against that diagnosis, and the mural nodule is generally highly vascular. Signal void from feeding vessels may also be seen on MRI. Ganglioglioma occurs in children and young adults, and is also a low-grade tumour. The temporal lobe is the most common site of the tumour, and patients usually present with seizures. These are generally cystic tumours without significant surrounding oedema. Mural nodules may be present.

CASE 5.6

Age: 39 years	Gender: Female
Clinical problem: Recurrent swelling and pain of the left submandibular region	
Images in exam case: CT (2), MRI (3)	

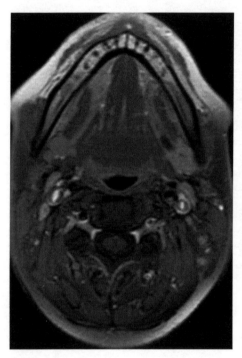

Figure 30a

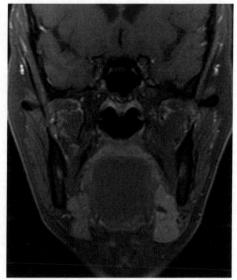

Figure 30b

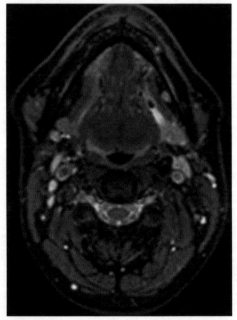

Figure 30c

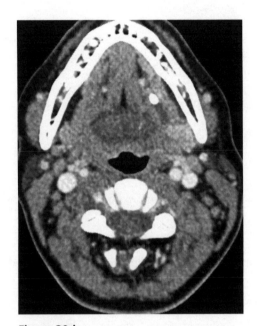

Figure 30d

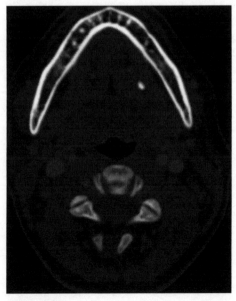

Figure 30e

FINDINGS

1. Post-contrast fat-suppressed T1 axial and coronal MRI:
   a. Enlarged left submandibular salivary gland
   b. Greater enhancement of the left submandibular gland in comparison with the right
   c. Dilated left Wharton's duct
   d. No focal mass or abscess.
2. STIR axial:
   a. Diffuse high signal within the enlarged left submandibular salivary gland
   b. Low-signal filling defect at the distal aspect of the left Wharton's duct with proximal dilatation.
3. CT neck:
   a. Enhancing diffusely enlarged left submandibular salivary gland with dilated Wharton's duct
   b. Calculus at the distal end of the left Wharton's duct.

DIAGNOSIS

Left submandibular sialadenitis secondary to obstructing submandibular duct calculus.

FURTHER INVESTIGATIONS AND MANAGEMENT

ENT referral for resection of submandibular duct calculus followed by sialodochoplasty.

FURTHER INFORMATION

The submandibular duct is the commonest site for salivary duct calculi, as the secretions are viscid and alkaline, and the duct courses 'uphill', predisposing to stasis. Sublingual and minor salivary gland calculi are extremely uncommon. Ductal strictures also predispose to calculus formation. Symptoms are recurrent pain and swelling exacerbated by eating. The obstructed gland becomes inflamed. CT is better for visualisation of calcified stones. Conventional or MR sialography can also diagnose salivary duct calculi.

Case bag 6

CASE 6.1

Age: 38 years	Gender: Female
Clinical problem: Headache and visual disturbance	
Images in exam case: MRI (5)	

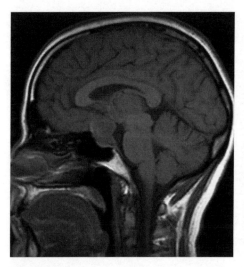

Figure 31a

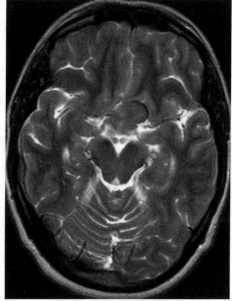

Figure 31b

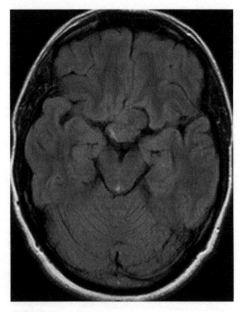

Figure 31c

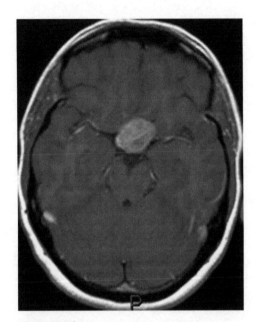

Figure 31d

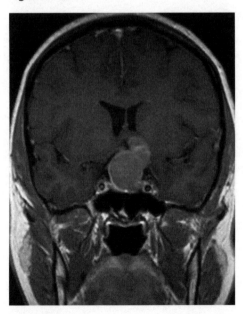

Figure 31e

FINDINGS

1. Pre-contrast T1 sagittal:
   a. Large mass arising from the pituitary fossa and extending into the suprasellar cistern
   b. Enlarged pituitary fossa.
2. T2 and FLAIR axial:
   a. Well-defined rounded mass in the suprasellar cistern
   b. Mass isointense to the grey matter
   c. Compression of the optic chiasm.
3. Post-contrast T1 coronal and axial images:
   a. Homogeneous enhancement of the mass
   b. No invasion into the cavernous sinuses
   c. Third ventricle displaced to the right.

MAIN DIAGNOSIS

Pituitary macroadenoma.

DIFFERENTIAL DIAGNOSIS

1. Craniopharyngioma. However, there is no suggestion of calcifications or cystic components.
2. Rathke's cleft cyst. However, there is solid homogeneous enhancement, which argues against this diagnosis.
3. Pituitary metastasis. However, there is no associated bone destruction and no adjacent brain parenchymal oedema.

FURTHER INVESTIGATIONS AND MANAGEMENT

1. Visual field assessment.
2. Neurosurgical referral with a view to trans-sphenoidal resection.

FURTHER INFORMATION

Pituitary macroadenomas are over 10 mm in diameter and are usually hormonally inactive. The mass can extend into the suprasellar cistern or into the cavernous sinuses. There is homogeneous enhancement of the mass following contrast administration. Focal areas of necrosis and haemorrhage can occur. Treatment with bromocriptine increases the risk of haemorrhage.

CASE 6.2

Age: 59 years	Gender: Female
Clinical problem: Shortness of breath	
Images in exam case: Plain radiograph (1), CT (3)	

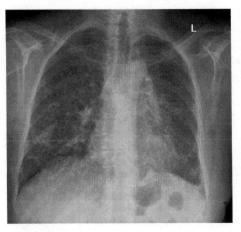

Figure 32a

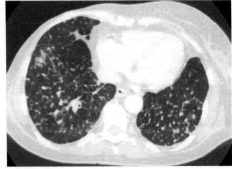

Figure 32b

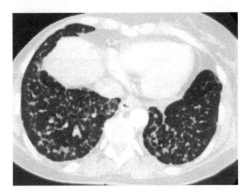

Figure 32c

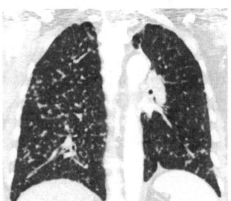

Figure 32d

FINDINGS

1. Chest X-ray:
   a. Diffuse nodularity throughout both lungs
   b. Previous right mastectomy. Surgical clips projected overlying the right lower chest
   c. Surgical clips projected adjacent to superior aspect of the left hilum. Elevated left hilum
   d. Left hemithorax volume loss, and loss of left heart border
   e. Blunting of left costophrenic angle.
2. CT thorax:
   a. Multiple small nodules throughout both lungs
   b. Interlobular septal thickening in the right lower lobe
   c. Previous right mastectomy.

INTERPRETATION

Diffuse bilateral pulmonary metastases with right lower lobe lymphangitic carcinomatosis on a background of previous left upper lobectomy and right mastectomy.

MAIN DIAGNOSIS

Metastatic breast carcinoma.

DIFFERENTIAL DIAGNOSIS

Metastatic lung carcinoma.

FURTHER INVESTIGATIONS AND MANAGEMENT

Oncology referral.

FURTHER INFORMATION

There was a history of treated cancers of breast and lung in this case, so metastatic disease of either cancer was possible. Pulmonary lymphangitic carcinomatosis occurs due to tumour growth in the pulmonary lymphatic system. Carcinomas of breast, lung, gastrointestinal tract, cervix and thyroid, and metastatic adenocarcinoma of unknown primary can all produce lymphangitic carcinomatosis. Interlobular septal thickening and nodularity, thickening of the peribronchovascular interstitium and subpleural nodularity are the features of this condition. There may also be associated lymph node enlargement and pleural effusions.

CASE 6.3

Age: 24 years	Gender: Male
Clinical problem: Gradual-onset sensory neural hearing loss and ataxia	
Images in exam case: MRI (4)	

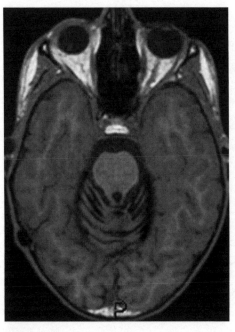

Figure 33a

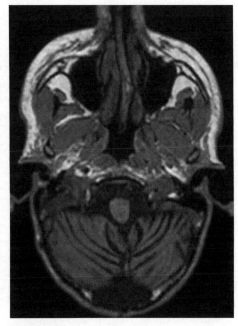

Figure 33b

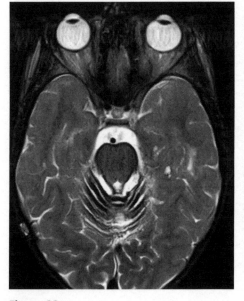

Figure 33c

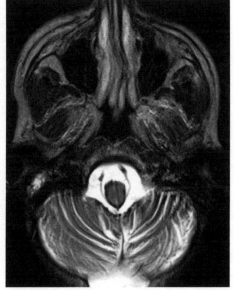

Figure 33d

FINDINGS

T1 and T2 axial images:
1. Marked low signal outlining the cerebellar folia – more pronounced on T2 than on T1 images
2. Low signal also outlining the brainstem
3. Defect of the occipital bone with posterior fossa meningocoele/ pseudomeningocoele.

DIAGNOSIS

Superficial siderosis of the CNS, most probably from previous posterior fossa surgery.

FURTHER INVESTIGATIONS AND MANAGEMENT

1. Determine the history of previous surgery.
2. Neurology referral.

FURTHER INFORMATION

Superficial siderosis of the CNS occurs as a result of chronic recurrent haemorrhage. Causes include dural arteriovenous malformations, tumours or previous CNS surgery. Sensorineural hearing loss, ataxia and multiple cranial nerve palsies are the usual presenting features. MRI shows a low-signal lining of haemosiderin over the brainstem, cerebellar folia and cranial nerves. This finding is most pronounced in gradient echo sequence, due to the susceptibility effects of haemosiderin.

CASE 6.4

Age: 45 years	Gender: Male
Clinical problem: Recovering right-sided weakness	
Images in exam case: MRI (4)	

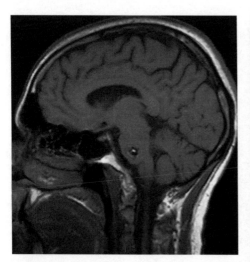

Figure 34a

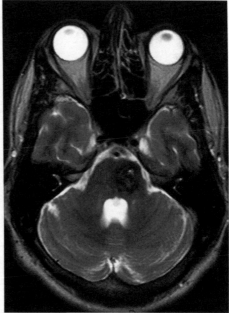

Figure 34b

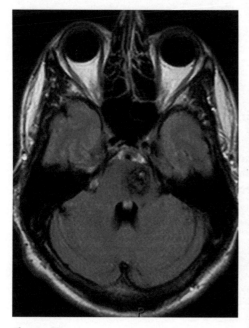

Figure 34c

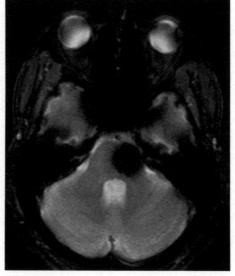

Figure 34d

FINDINGS

1. T1 sagittal MRI:
   a. Pontine mass with central high signal surrounded by a continuous low-signal rim.
2. T2/FLAIR axial MRI:
   a. The mass arises from the left side of the pons. The signal is mixed but predominantly low.
3. GRE T2 MRI:
   a. Marked low signal with blooming artefact, consistent with haemosiderin rim.

INTERPRETATION

Mixed-signal pontine mass with haemosiderin rim.

MAIN DIAGNOSIS

Cavernous haemangioma arising from the left side of the pons.

DIFFERENTIAL DIAGNOSIS

1. Previous simple pontine haemorrhage. However, this would leave a residual 'slit-like' cavity rather than a rounded mass.
2. Haemorrhagic neoplasm. However, these tend to have an incomplete haemosiderin ring.

FURTHER INVESTIGATIONS AND MANAGEMENT

1. Review of previous imaging if available.
2. Neurosurgical referral.

FURTHER INFORMATION

Cavernous haemangiomas are typically described as 'mulberry-like' lesions on MRI. This is due to previous haemorrhages of different ages. Infratentorial cavernomas are more likely to bleed than supratentorial ones. Multiple cavernous haemangiomas tend to be familial. Previous spontaneous haemorrhage would result in a slit-like cavity rather than a rounded mass. Haemorrhagic neoplasms do not usually have a complete rim of haemosiderin. Gradient echo images demonstrate the 'blooming' artefact from susceptibility effects of haemosiderin.

CASE 6.5

Age: 70 years	Gender: Male
Clinical problem: Weight loss	
Images in exam case: CT (7)	

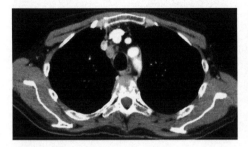

Figure 35a

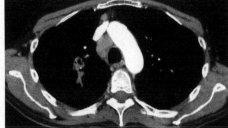

Figure 35b

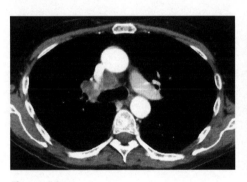

Figure 35c

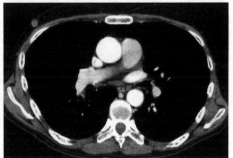

Figure 35d

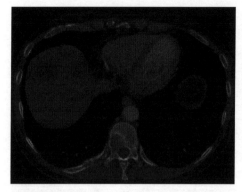

Figure 35e

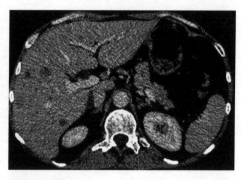

Figure 35f

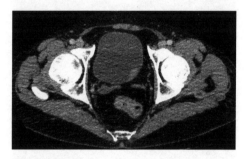

Figure 35g

FINDINGS

1. CT thorax, abdomen and pelvis:
   a. Right upper lobe cavitating mass
   b. Right hilar, right paratracheal, precarinal and prevascular lymph node enlargement
   c. Thoracic vertebral body destruction associated with a soft tissue mass
   d. Right-sided posterior rib destruction
   e. Subcutaneous soft tissue nodule in the right anterior chest wall
   f. Multiple low-attenuation liver lesions
   g. Enhancing nodule arising from the left side of the urinary bladder wall.

MAIN DIAGNOSIS

1. Right upper lobe bronchogenic carcinoma with lymph node, liver, subcutaneous and bone metastases.
2. Incidental transitional-cell carcinoma (TCC) of the urinary bladder.

DIFFERENTIAL DIAGNOSIS

Transitional-cell carcinoma of the bladder with lung, lymph node, bone, liver and subcutaneous metastases. However, the distribution of lymph node disease is more suggestive of primary bronchogenic carcinoma.

FURTHER INVESTIGATIONS AND MANAGEMENT

1. Biopsy of subcutaneous nodule for tissue diagnosis.
2. Urology referral for cystoscopy and biopsy.
3. Respiratory/urology MDT discussion.

FURTHER INFORMATION

Most lung cancers drain into the ipsilateral hilar lymph node before reaching the mediastinum. However, sometimes particularly the upper lobe tumours may bypass the hilar lymph nodes and reach the mediastinum.

More than 90% of the bladder tumours are transitional-cell carcinomas (TCC). Adenocarcinomas are associated with patent urachus. Almost a third of the patients have multifocal disease at presentation. External iliac followed by common iliac and para-aortic lymph nodes can become involved with bladder cancers. Mediastinal lymph nodes may subsequently become enlarged.

CASE 6.6

Age: 25 years	Gender: Female
Clinical problem: Back pain	
Images in exam case: MRI (5)	

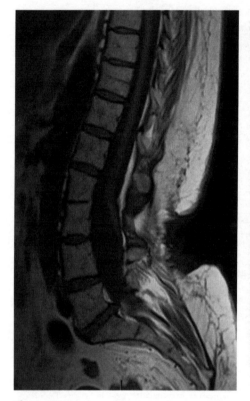 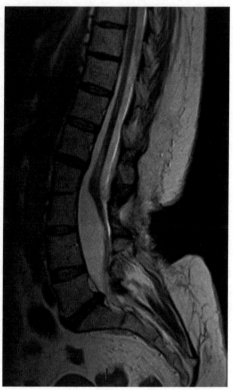

Figure 36a　　　　　　　　　**Figure 36b**

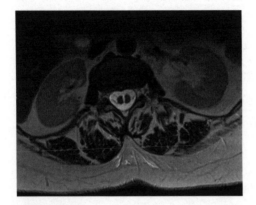

Figure 36c

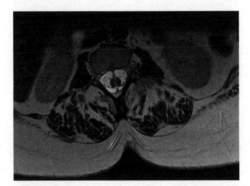

Figure 36d

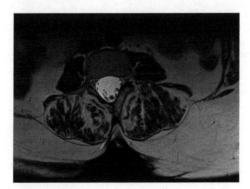

Figure 36e

FINDINGS

1. T1 and T2 sagittals:
   a. Low-lying, tethered spinal cord with the conus lying at the level of the lower border of the L3 vertebra
   b. L2/3 congenital block vertebra
   c. Enlarged lumbar thecal sac
   d. L5/S1 intervertebral disc bulge
   e. Defect in the posterior subcutaneous fat.
2. T2 axials:
   a. Split spinal cord
   b. Low-signal septum between the two hemicords
   c. Thickened filum terminale
   d. Deficient posterior right lamina at the level of defect in the posterior subcutaneous fat
   e. Normal kidneys.

DIAGNOSIS

1. Diastomatomyelia.
2. Spina bifida occulta.
3. Congenital block vertebra L2/3.
4. L5/S1 disc bulge.

FURTHER INVESTIGATIONS AND MANAGEMENT

1. MR skull base to assess for Chiari malformation.
2. Evaluation of the cervicothoracic spinal cord to assess the superior extent of diastomatomyelia and to look for a hydromyelic cavity.

FURTHER INFORMATION

Diastomatomyelia is a longitudinal split in the spinal cord. There may be two separate dural sacs or a single large dural sac. The two hemicords may be separated by a bony or cartilaginous spur or a fibrous band. The hemicords may unite below the cleft. It is largely associated with spinal anomalies such as spina bifida, hemivertebrae or scoliosis. Tethered cord, meningomyelocoele, Chiari II malformations and syringohydromyelia are other associations. Congenital block vertebrae have typical wasting at the intervertebral level. Post-inflammatory vertebral fusion does not have such wasting. Normal filum terminale is less than 2 mm thick.

Case bag 7

CASE 7.1

Age: 73 years	Gender: Male
Clinical problem: Rectal bleeding	
Images in exam case: MRI (4)	

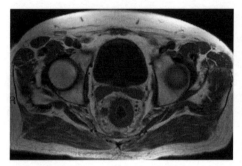

Figure 37a

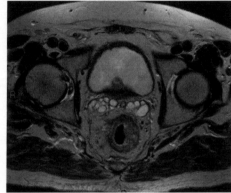

Figure 37b

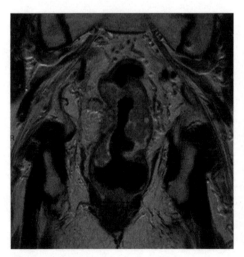

Figure 37c

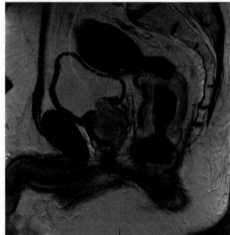

Figure 37d

FINDINGS

1. T1 axial:
   a. Marked circumferential rectal wall thickening consistent with rectal carcinoma
   b. Irregularity of the mesorectal fat adjacent to the rectal wall towards the right, consistent with mesorectal fat invasion
   c. Enlarged mesorectal lymph node to the right of the rectum. The node is in proximity to the mesorectal fascia, but there is no evidence of mesorectal fascial invasion.
2. T2 axial, coronal and sagittal:
   a. The tumour is well above the level of the plane of the anal sphincters
   b. Enlarged prostate with trabeculated bladder wall.

DIAGNOSIS

1. Rectal carcinoma, local stage T3N1.
2. Benign prostatic hypertrophy.

FURTHER INVESTIGATIONS AND MANAGEMENT

1. CT scan of chest and abdomen for completion of staging.
2. Sigmoidoscopy and biopsy of tumour if these have not already been performed.
3. Surgical referral for tumour resection.

FURTHER INFORMATION

Rectal cancer staging is done by MRI for local staging and CT chest, abdomen and pelvis for distant disease. Total mesorectal excision (TME) involves the resection of tumour and the surrounding mesorectal fat, and is the treatment of choice. It is important to identify whether or not the mesorectal fascia is invaded, as this has a bearing on how these patients will be treated. Those without mesorectal fascial invasion undergo surgery directly, whereas those with mesorectal fascial invasion undergo radiotherapy prior to surgery to encourage tumour regression. However, the disease is still T3, irrespective of whether the mesorectal fascia is invaded. It is also important to give an idea of how close the tumour is to the mesorectal fascia.

CASE 7.2

Age: 58 years	Gender: Female
Clinical problem: Partial seizures	
Images in exam case: Plain radiograph (1), CT (7)	

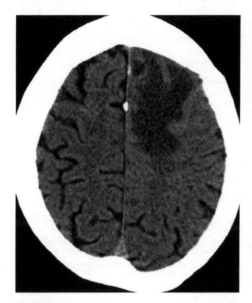

Figure 38a

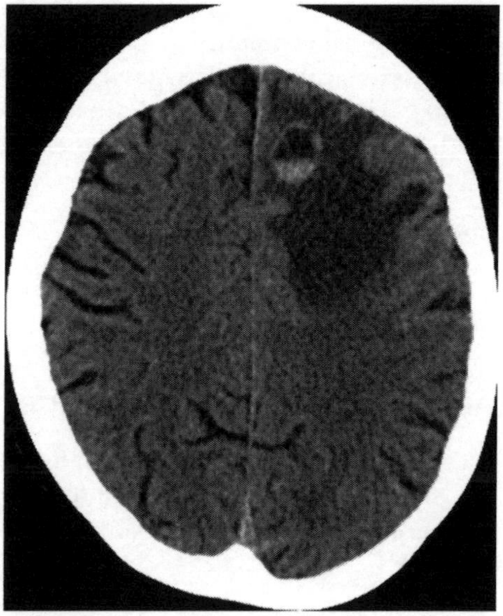

Figure 38b

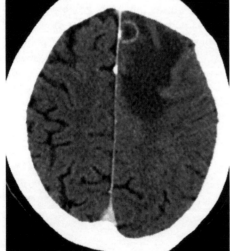

Figure 38c

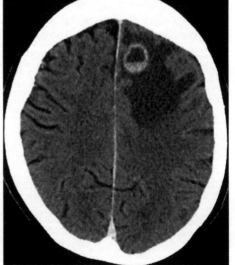

Figure 38d

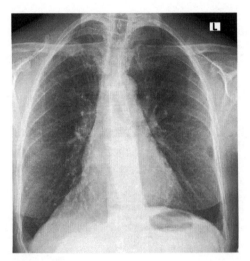

Figure 38e

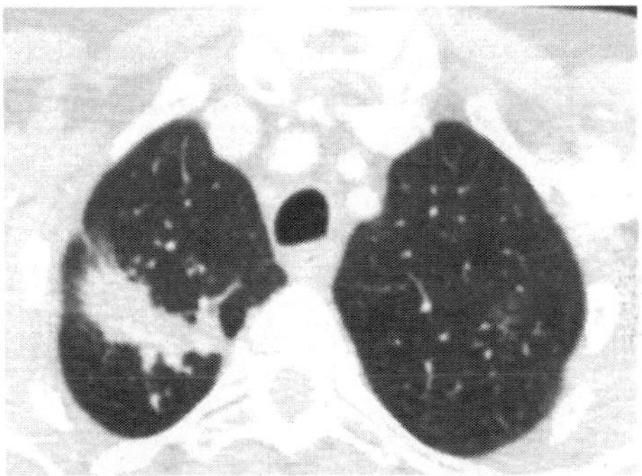

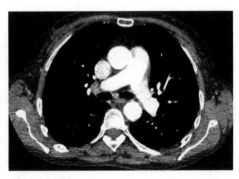

Figure 38f

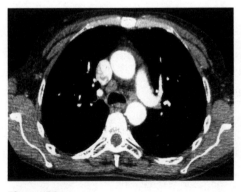

Figure 38g

Figure 38h

FINDINGS

1. CT brain pre- and post-contrast images:
   a. Two left frontal ring-enhancing masses in the parafalcine location
   b. Extensive white matter oedema
   c. Mass effect causing local sulcal effacement
   d. Larger lesion contains fluid-fluid level in pre-contrast image, suggestive of haemorrhage within it.
2. Chest X-ray:
   a. Ill-defined right apical opacification
   b. Adjacent pleural thickening and pleural tenting but no clear bone destruction
   c. No other lesion.
3. CT thorax:
   a. Right upper lobe spiculated mass
   b. Adjacent pleural thickening
   c. Right hilar and precarinal lymph node enlargement.

INTERPRETATION

Spiculated right upper lobe lung mass and left frontal ring-enhancing lesions, one of which has internal haemorrhage.

MAIN DIAGNOSIS

Bronchogenic carcinoma with right hilar and mediastinal lymph node enlargement and cerebral metastases.

DIFFERENTIAL DIAGNOSIS

Right apical tuberculosis with caseating tubercular granulomas of the brain. However, the lesion has the typical spiculated appearance of a bronchogenic carcinoma.

FURTHER INVESTIGATIONS AND MANAGEMENT

1. Neurology referral for immediate management of complications arising from the brain metastases.
2. Completion of staging by performing CT upper abdomen.
3. Percutaneous biopsy of lung lesion.
4. Lung cancer MDT referral for further management decisions.

FURTHER INFORMATION

Metastases are the most common supratentorial masses in adults. The primary tumour may arise from lung, breast, melanoma, gastrointestinal tract, kidney or thyroid. Metastases tend to occur at the grey–white matter junction, and more commonly in the anterior circulation than the posterior one. Metastases have sharper, better defined borders than gliomas, and the vasogenic oedema is generally out of proportion to the size of the metastases. Cerebral metastases that are prone to haemorrhage arise from malignant melanoma, choriocarcinoma, bronchogenic carcinoma, renal-cell carcinoma or thyroid carcinoma.

CASE 7.3

Age: 46 years	Gender: Female
Clinical problem: Pain on left side of the neck with left arm weakness	
Images in exam case: CT (1), MRI (9)	

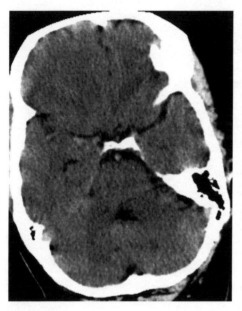

Figure 39a

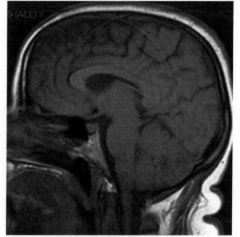

Figure 39b

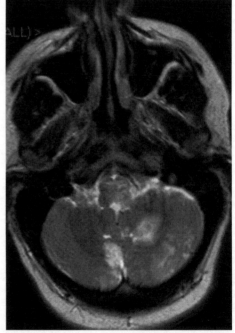

Figure 39c

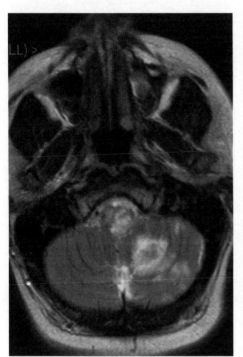

Figure 39d

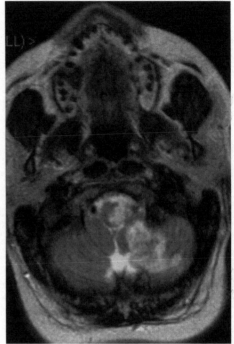

Figure 39e

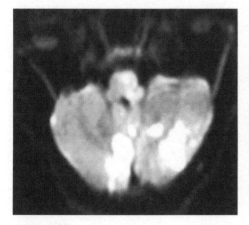

Figure 39f

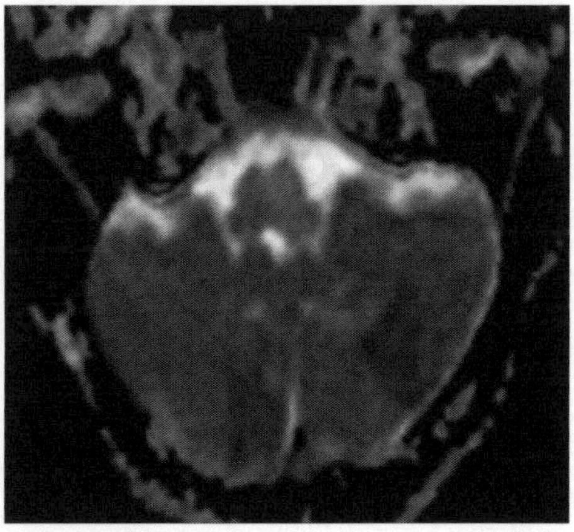

Figure 39g

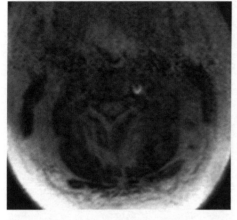

Figure 39h

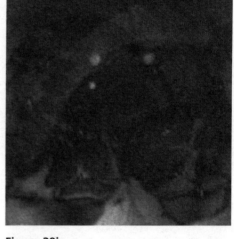

Figure 39i

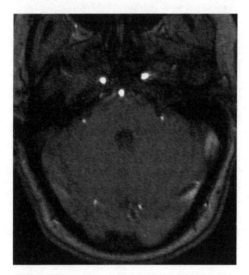

Figure 39j

FINDINGS

1. Non-contrast CT brain:
   a. Normal.
2. T1-weighted MRI:
   a. Low signal extending out to the peripheral cortex in the posterior inferior aspect of the left side of the cerebellum
   b. Cerebellar sulcal effacement in the affected areas.
3. T2-weighted MRI:
   a. High signal in the medulla, pons and inferior cerebellum bilaterally, but more extensive on the left side
   b. Loss of normal flow void in the left vertebral artery.
4. DWI and ADC maps:
   a. High signal in the medulla, pons and inferior cerebellum bilaterally with corresponding low signal on ADC maps, consistent with diffusion restriction.
5. Fat-suppressed T1 images through the upper neck:
   a. Crescentic high signal at the posterior aspect of the left vertebral artery, consistent with intramural haematoma.
6. MR angiogram neck:
   a. Non-visualisation of the left vertebral artery
   b. Other vessels normal.

DIAGNOSIS

1. Left vertebral artery dissection.
2. Bilateral posterior circulation infarction, more extensive on the left side, affecting the pons, medulla and inferior cerebellum.

FURTHER MANAGEMENT

1. Urgent neurology referral for anticoagulation to prevent recurrent embolic events.
2. Neurointervention consultation for potential stenting.

FURTHER INFORMATION

Vertebral artery dissections most commonly present as headache and neck pain followed by posterior circulation ischaemia. Vertebral artery dissection can be extradural, intradural, or extradural extending intradurally. Intradural vertebral dissection presents with either ischaemic symptoms or subarachnoid haemorrhage. Extradural dissection usually presents with neck pain and posterior circulation ischaemia. Patients with extracranial dissections are anticoagulated to prevent thrombosis and embolism. Subacute intramural haematoma is best visualised on fat-suppressed T1-weighted MRI as a crescent of high signal surrounding an eccentric flow void.

CASE 7.4

Age: 30 years	Gender: Male
Clinical problem: Knee injury followed by swelling	
Images in exam case: MRI (5)	

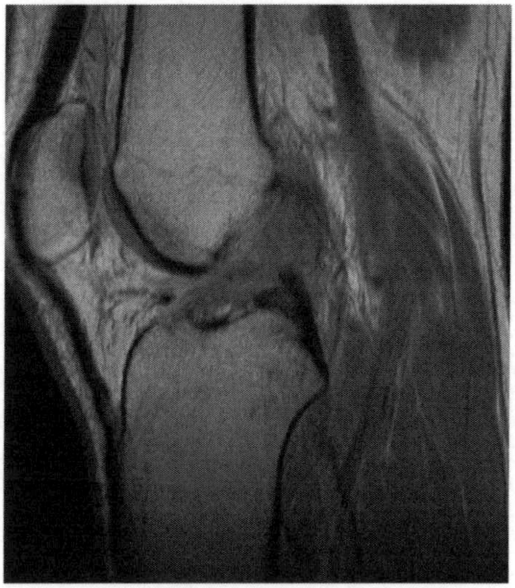

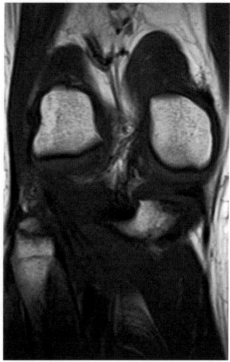

Figure 40a

Figure 40b

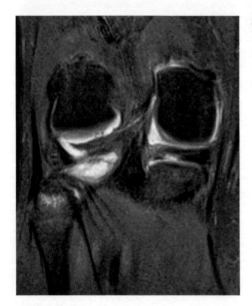

Figure 40c

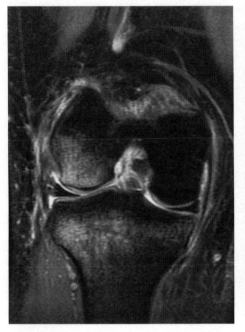

Figure 40d

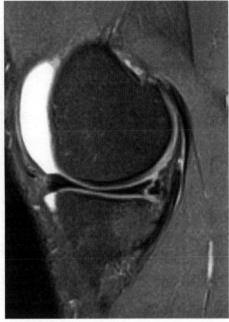

Figure 40e

FINDINGS

1. PD sagittal:
   a. No visible fibres of anterior cruciate ligament, consistent with complete ACL rupture.
2. T1 and PD fat-saturated coronal:
   a. Low-signal fracture line through the head of fibula associated with adjacent bone marrow oedema
   b. Bone oedema of the lateral femoral condyle and lateral tibial plateau
   c. Fluid signal within, outside and inside the lateral collateral ligament, consistent with lateral collateral ligament tear
   d. Fluid signal outside and inside the medial collateral ligament, consistent with partial tear/sprain of the medial collateral ligament.
3. PD fat-saturated sagittal:
   a. Vertical tear of the posterior third of the medial meniscus
   b. Knee joint effusion.

DIAGNOSIS

Complex injury involving arcuate complex avulsion fracture of the fibular styloid associated with complete ACL rupture, vertical tear of the medial meniscus and injury of the medial and lateral collateral ligaments.

FURTHER INVESTIGATIONS AND MANAGEMENT

Urgent orthopaedic referral for further management, as these injuries can lead to chronic knee instability.

FURTHER INFORMATION

Like Segond fracture, arcuate complex avulsion fracture can appear subtle on plain radiographs and can be associated with significant soft tissue injuries. The arcuate complex consists of posterolateral knee-stabilising structures such as the lateral collateral ligament, biceps femoris tendon, popliteus muscle and tendon and adjacent ligaments. The fracture line is oriented horizontally.

CASE 7.5

Age: 5 years	Gender: Male
Clinical problem: Recurrent chest infections	
Images in exam case: Plain radiograph (1), CT (3)	

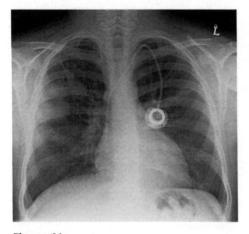

Figure 41a

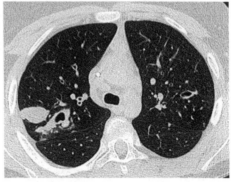

Figure 41b

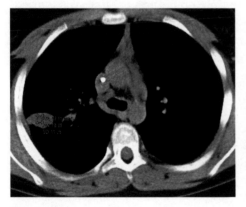

Figure 41c

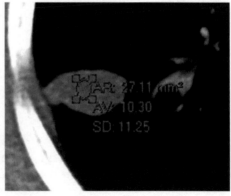

Figure 41d

FINDINGS

1. CXR:
   a. Portacath *in situ* with tip projecting over the right atrium
   b. Three ovoid opacities are projected over the right mid zone
   c. No evidence of cavitation.
2. CT:
   a. Bronchial dilatation and wall thickening in both upper lobes
   b. The CXR opacities correspond to fluid density structures related to a dilated thickened right upper lobe bronchus
   c. No cavitation, and no surrounding ground glass halo
   d. No mediastinal adenopathy on the selected slices.

INTERPRETATION

Fluid-filled cystic spaces in relation to dilated thickened bronchi in the upper lobes in a young patient.

MAIN DIAGNOSIS

Right upper lobe mucocoeles on a background of cystic fibrosis.

DIFFERENTIAL DIAGNOSIS

Aspergillosis. However, this is unlikely as there are no features of intracavitary mycetoma or invasive aspergillosis.

FURTHER INVESTIGATIONS AND MANAGEMENT

Respiratory team review.

FURTHER INFORMATION

Bronchial mucocoele (bronchocoele) is due to sterile fluid accumulation distal to an obstructed bronchus. Apart from cystic fibrosis, where the bronchi can be obstructed secondary to viscid secretions, bronchopulmonary aspergillosis, obstructing tumours such as carcinoids, and congenital bronchial atresia can also give rise to bronchocoeles.

CASE 7.6

Age: 7 years	Gender: Male
Clinical problem: Abdominal pain	
Images in exam case: Ultrasound (3), CT (3)	

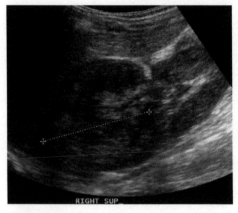

Figure 42a

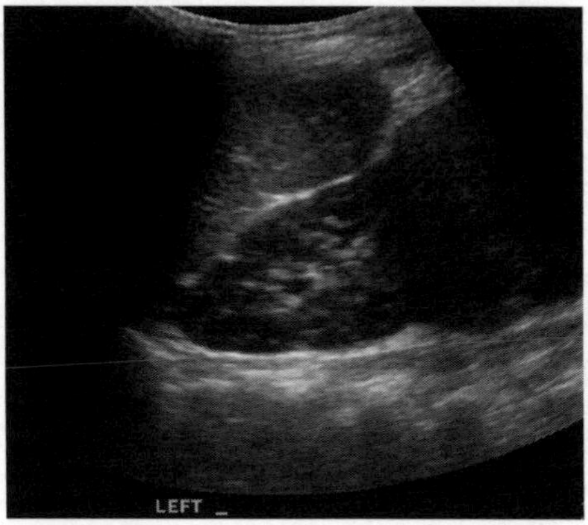

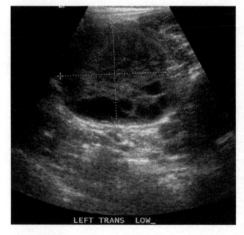

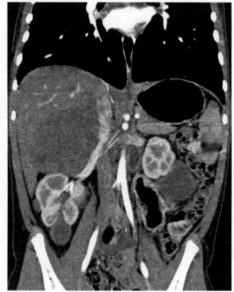

Figure 42b

Figure 42c

Figure 42d

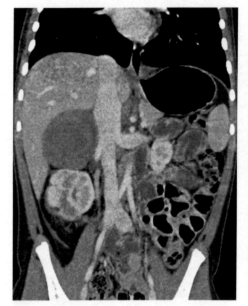

Figure 42e

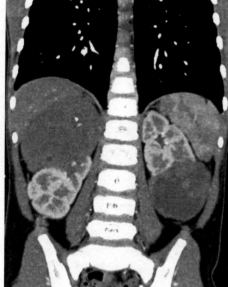

Figure 42f

FINDINGS

1. USS:
   a. Large, heterogenous but predominantly hypoechoic mass arising from the upper pole of the right kidney
   b. A further large hypoechoic mass arising from the lower pole of the left kidney. Cystic areas within the mass
   c. No hydronephrosis.
2. CT:
   a. Large, well-circumscribed exophytic mass arising from the right upper renal pole. Flecks of central calcifications. The rest of the kidney is displaced inferiorly
   b. Two smaller exophytic lesions arising from the lower pole of the right kidney
   c. Large heterogenous mass arising from the left lower renal pole
   d. All lesions enhance poorly in comparison with the renal parenchyma
   e. No renal vein invasion on either side. The right renal vein is displaced and attenuated
   f. No lymph node enlargement
   g. No mass in the visualised liver.

INTERPRETATION

Bilateral well-defined heterogeneous renal masses with the right renal mass displacing the right renal vein.

MAIN DIAGNOSIS

Bilateral Wilms' tumour – no vascular invasion, no nodal disease or liver metastasis.

DIFFERENTIAL DIAGNOSIS

Neuroblastoma. However, these tend to cross the midline and encase vessels rather than displace them.

FURTHER INVESTIGATIONS AND MANAGEMENT

1. CT thorax to exclude pulmonary metastases.
2. Referral to paediatric oncology and surgical services for surgery and chemotherapy.

FURTHER INFORMATION

Wilms' tumour is the most common renal tumour in children. The peak age is 2–4 years. Wilms' tumour can be bilateral in 5–10% of cases. Several congenital malformations such as hemihypertrophy, cerebral gigantism, Beckwith–Wiedemann syndrome, neurofibromatosis, and horseshoe and duplex kidney can be associated with Wilms' tumour. Bilateral renal tumours make this a stage V tumour. Tumour calcifications occur in only 10% of cases.

Neuroblastoma is the commonest abdominal tumour in infants, and the second commonest tumour in children (after Wilms' tumour). Small calcifications are typical. Encasement of an adjacent vessel is a characteristic imaging feature. Intraspinal extension through neural foramina can also occur. Metastases are most commonly to the bone, whereas the lungs are the commonest site of metastasis from Wilms' tumour.

Case bag 8

CASE 8.1

Age: 3 years	Gender: Male
Clinical problem: Leg spasticity. Previous cardiac surgery. The patient's mother is diabetic	
Images in exam case: MRI (5)	

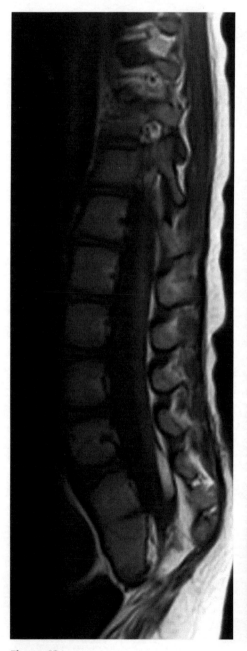 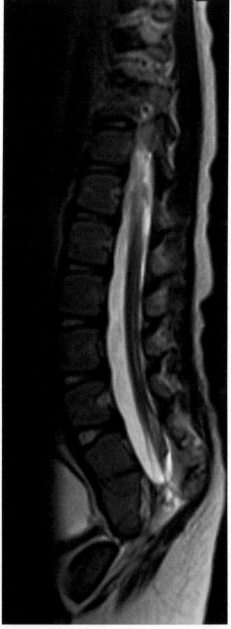

Figure 43a   **Figure 43b**

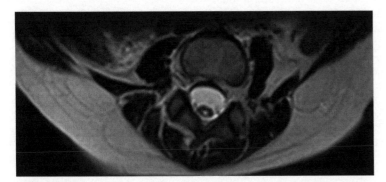

Figure 43c

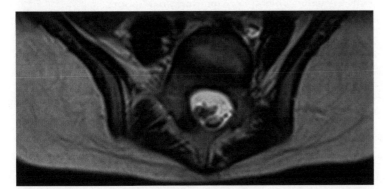

Figure 43d

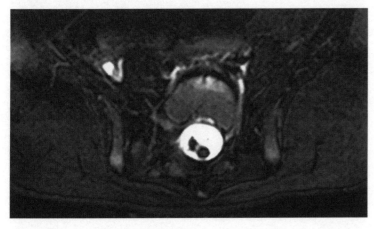

Figure 43e

FINDINGS

1. T1- and T2-weighted sagittal images:
    a. Incomplete formation of the sacrum, with partial fusion of L5–S1
    b. Spinal cord tethered down to the level of L5
    c. Linear T1 and T2 high-signal mass attached to the posterior aspect of the distal spinal cord
    d. Dilated central canal of the distal spinal cord.
2. T2 and STIR axial images:
    a. Dilated central canal at L4 level
    b. Irregular T2 high-signal mass attached to the cord at L5 level, which loses signal on STIR image, consistent with a fatty mass.

INTERPRETATION

Incomplete formation of lower sacrum. Fatty mass attached to the tip of the low-lying tethered cord, consistent with a spinal cord lipoma. Terminal hydromyelia.

DIAGNOSIS

Caudal regression syndrome with tethered cord and terminal lipoma.

FURTHER INVESTIGATIONS AND MANAGEMENT

Previous cardiac surgery in this case suggests pre-existing cardiac anomalies. Examination of the renal tract is required if it has not already been performed, as caudal regression syndrome may be associated with VACTERL anomalies.

FURTHER INFORMATION

Caudal regression syndrome, also called sacral agenesis, is most commonly seen in children with diabetic mothers. The characteristic finding is a wedge-shaped or blunt-ended high-lying spinal cord with distal hypoplasia. Sometimes the cord may be low and tethered, and a lipomeningocele may be associated with it.

CASE 8.2

Age: 6 years	Gender: Female
Clinical problem: History of 1 week of coryzal symptoms and 2 days of arm and leg paraesthesia	
Images in exam case: MRI (11)	

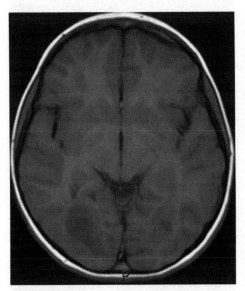

Figure 44a

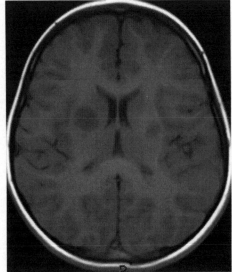

Figure 44b

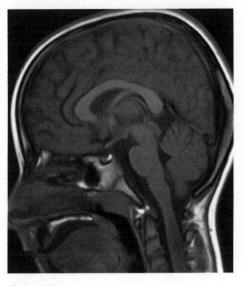

Figure 44c

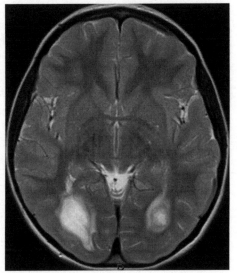

Figure 44d

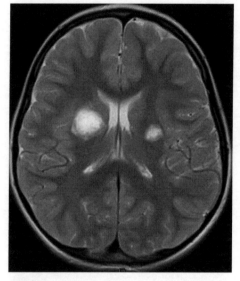

Figure 44e

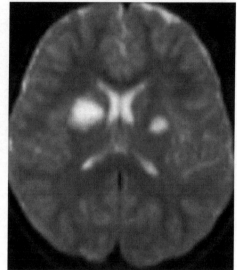

Figure 44f

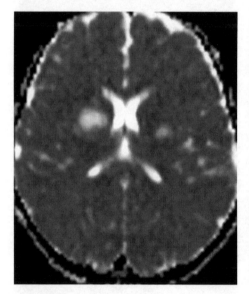

Figure 44g

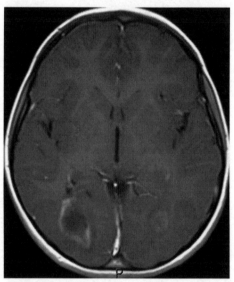

Figure 44h

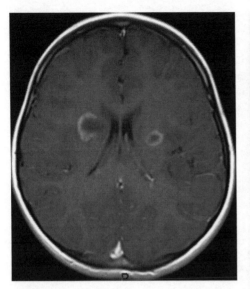

Figure 44i

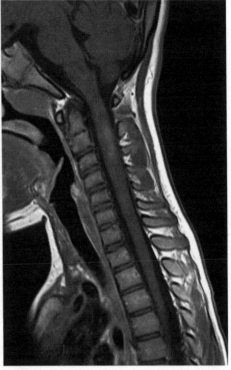

Figure 44j

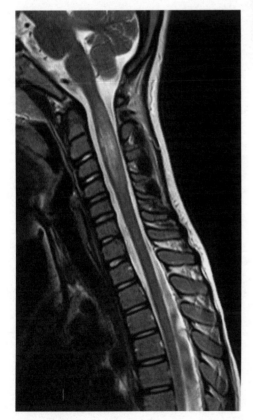

Figure 44k

FINDINGS

1. MRI brain:
   a. Multiple symmetrically distributed T1 low-signal and T2 high-signal white matter lesions in each of the parietal and occipital lobes
   b. Mild surrounding vasogenic oedema
   c. Peripheral enhancement in an 'incomplete ring' pattern
   d. No diffusion restriction.
2. MRI cervical spinal cord:
   a. Expansile lesion within the cervical cord, extending from the upper border of C2 to the upper border of C5
   b. Similar signal characteristics to brain lesions.

INTERPRETATION

Symmetrical T2 hyperintense peripherally enhancing lesions in the brain and spinal cord in a child with a recent history of coryzal symptoms.

MAIN DIAGNOSIS

Acute disseminated encephalomyelitis (ADEM).

DIFFERENTIAL DIAGNOSIS

Multiple sclerosis, with a relapsing remitting course.

FURTHER INVESTIGATIONS AND MANAGEMENT

1. Imaging of the rest of the spine is indicated.
2. Urgent neurology referral for CSF study and steroid therapy.

FURTHER INFORMATION

ADEM is a monophasic demyelinating disease with a self-limiting course. There is generally a history of recent viral infection or vaccination. ADEM is most frequently associated with varicella (chickenpox) infections, but may also follow rubella, mumps, influenza, infectious mononucleosis and *Mycoplasma* infections. Neurological symptoms and signs present late in the viral illness. Seizures are frequent. Diagnosis is established by a combination of CSF study and MRI in a patient who presents with a prodrome of viral illness. Without the history of preceding viral infection or immunisation, it may not be possible to distinguish ADEM from acute multiple sclerosis.

CASE 8.3

Age: 6 months	Gender: Male
Clinical problem: Distress and abdominal guarding	
Images in exam case: Ultrasound (4), plain radiograph (1)	

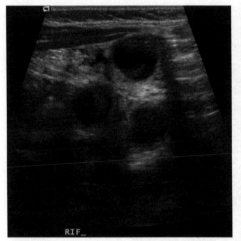

Figure 45a

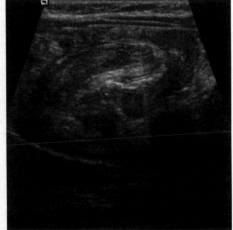

Figure 45b

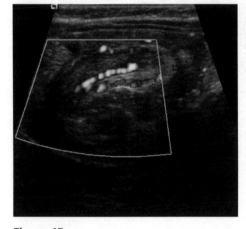

Figure 45c

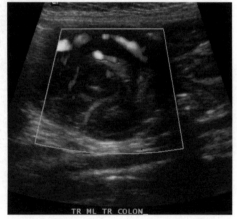

Figure 45d

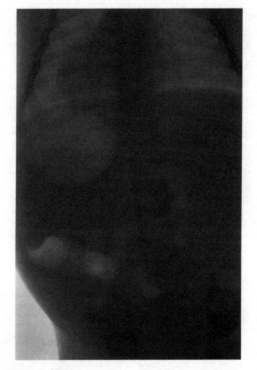

Figure 45e

FINDINGS

1. US abdomen:
   a. A mass showing the 'target sign' is seen in the left upper quadrant with alternating hypo- and hyperechoic layers. Appearances are consistent with intussusception
   b. Colour Doppler demonstrates flow within mesenteric vessels of the intussusceptum wall
   c. Dilated bowel loops in the right iliac fossa with a trace of free fluid.
2. Abdomen X-ray:
   a. The intussusceptum is seen as a soft tissue mass with an overlying crescent of gas in the left upper quadrant (meniscus sign)
   b. Distended gas-filled small bowel loops
   c. No free gas.

DIAGNOSIS

Ileo-ileocolic intussusception.

FURTHER INVESTIGATIONS AND MANAGEMENT

1. Pneumatic reduction.
2. If the latter is unsuccessful, surgical referral for operative treatment.

FURTHER INFORMATION

Intussusception in young children is usually due to lymphoid hyperplasia as a result of viral infections. Thus mesenteric lymph nodes may sometimes be seen. Other causes include Meckel's diverticulum, enteric duplication cysts, lymphoma, polyps or cystic fibrosis. In older children, intussusception can be a complication of Henoch–Schönlein purpura (HSP). The vast majority of intussusceptions occur in the ileocaecal region. Ultrasound is very sensitive and is the investigation of choice. On axial images it gives the 'bull's eye' (or 'target') appearance, and on longitudinal images the 'pseudokidney' sign is observed. A Doppler signal is detected from the mesenteric vasculature between the various layers of the bowel wall. Bowel proximal to the intussusception is dilated. There may sometimes be fluid between the layers of bowel wall. Free intraperitoneal fluid may also be present. Pneumatic reduction (approximately 120 mmHg pressure) under fluoroscopic control is the treatment of choice. Perforation is an absolute contraindication to pneumatic reduction.

CASE 8.4

Age: 9 years	Gender: Male
Clinical problem: Headaches and visual disturbance	
Images in exam case: CT (1), MRI (5)	

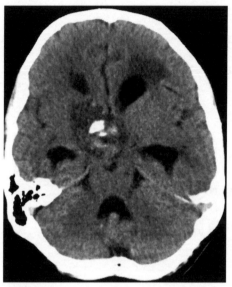

Figure 46a

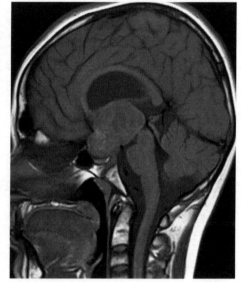

Figure 46b

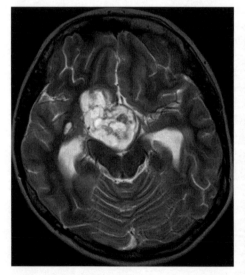

Figure 46c

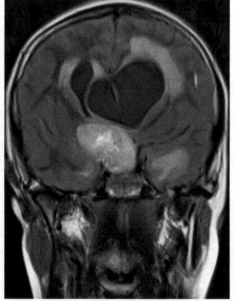

Figure 46d

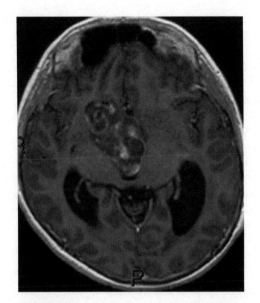

Figure 46e

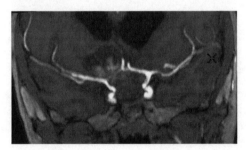

Figure 46f

FINDINGS

1. Non-contrast CT:
   a. Heterogeneous suprasellar mass containing coarse calcifications
   b. Associated hydrocephalus
   c. Low attenuation adjacent to frontal horns of the lateral ventricles, consistent with transependymal CSF flow.
2. MRI:
   a. T1 sagittal: large intermediate-signal dumb-bell-shaped suprasellar mass. The pituitary gland is separate from the mass, but is compressed at the inferior aspect of the sella turcica. Normal aqueduct and fourth ventricle
   b. T2 axial: the mass has a heterogeneous high signal with areas of low signal within it. The cerebral peduncles are displaced posteriorly. The mass extends towards the right of the midline
   c. FLAIR coronal: the mass has a heterogeneous high signal. The optic chiasm cannot be identified separately, but is likely to be compressed. Cavernous sinuses are not invaded by the mass
   d. Post-contrast T1 axial: heterogenous rim and nodular enhancement, which suggests that there is a predominantly cystic component to the mass
   e. MRA: the mass encases and attenuates the A1 segment of the right anterior cerebral artery.

INTERPRETATION

Partly calcified mixed solid and cystic enhancing suprasellar mass causing obstructive hydrocephalus by compressing the third ventricle.

MAIN DIAGNOSIS

Craniopharyngioma.

DIFFERENTIAL DIAGNOSIS

1. Rathke's cleft cyst. However, most of these are homogeneous with no calcification or solid nodular enhancement.
2. Suprasellar meningioma. However, the age of the patient and the predominant cystic components argue against this diagnosis.

FURTHER INVESTIGATIONS AND MANAGEMENT

Neurosurgical referral.

FURTHER INFORMATION

Craniopharyngioma has a bimodal age distribution, usually occurring in children and adolescents, and having a second peak in the fifth decade of life.

The three hallmarks of craniopharyngioma are calcification, cyst formation and enhancement. CT is more sensitive than MRI for detection of calcifications, but MRI gives better evaluation of the extent and its relationship to the optic chiasm and pituitary gland. As the cysts may have haemorrhagic and proteinaceous contents, they may give a high signal intensity on T1.

CASE 8.5

Age: 75 years	Gender: Male
Clinical problem: Grumbling abdominal pain of 2-week duration following ERCP	
Images in exam case: Plain radiograph (1), CT (7)	

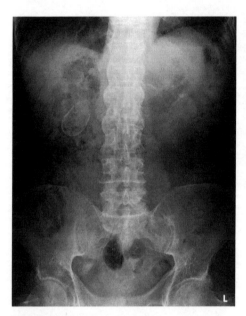

Figure 47a

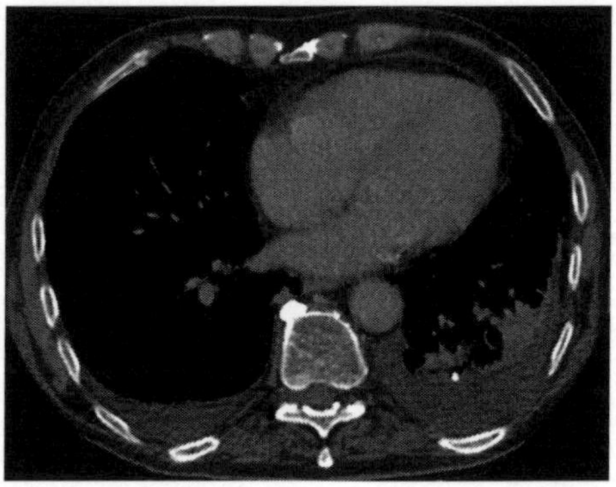

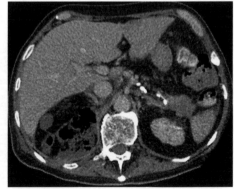

Figure 47b

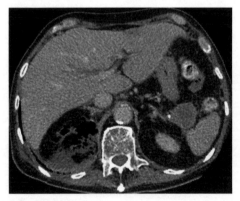

Figure 47c

Figure 47d

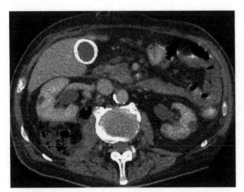

Figure 47e

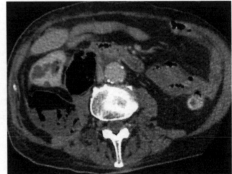

Figure 47f

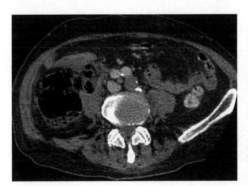

Figure 47g

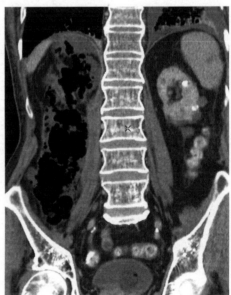

Figure 47h

FINDINGS

1. X-ray abdomen:
   a. Bubbly lucencies extending from the right subdiaphragmatic region down to the right iliac fossa. These do not appear intraluminal
   b. Loss of the right psoas shadow
   c. Curvilinear calcification in the right upper quadrant, probably due to calcified gallbladder wall
   d. Vascular calcifications along the splenic artery distribution
   e. Lumbar spine degenerative changes with osteophytic lipping.
2. CT abdomen:
   a. Large gas-containing right retroperitoneal collection extending from the right subdiaphragmatic region down into the right iliac fossa. The collection is medially related to the second part of the duodenum
   b. The collection displaces the right kidney anteriorly
   c. Low-attenuation mass related to the pancreatic tail
   d. Splenic artery calcification
   e. Ill-defined low-attenuation splenic lesion extending to the capsule, probably a splenic infarct
   f. Porcelain gallbladder
   g. Bilateral renal cysts
   h. Bibasal pleural effusions
   i. Left lower lobe consolidation and calcified granuloma.

INTERPRETATION

Right retroperitoneal gas- and fluid-containing collection related to the duodenum and a low-attenuation pancreatic tail mass.

MAIN DIAGNOSIS

1. Retroperitoneal abscess which is probably a complication of recent ERCP causing duodenal perforation.
2. Pancreatic tail mass, most probably an incidental primary pancreatic tumour.

DIFFERENTIAL DIAGNOSIS OF PANCREATIC MASS

Pancreatic pseudocyst. However, lack of peripancreatic inflammatory stranding and pancreatic parenchymal calcifications makes post-pancreatitis pseudocyst less likely.

FURTHER INVESTIGATIONS AND MANAGEMENT

1. Urgent surgical referral for management of right retroperitoneal abscess.
2. Follow-up of the pancreatic lesion once the patient's clinical condition has improved.

FURTHER INFORMATION

On plain radiograph, intra-abdominal abscesses may be seen as soft tissue density masses causing displacement of adjacent structures or obliteration of normal fat planes. Gas-containing abscesses give rise to a mottled appearance (resembling tiny bubbles) or sometimes a gas-fluid level. Intra-abdominal collections arise from appendicitis, cholecystitis, diverticulitis or perforated ulcers, or from recent laparotomy. Retroperitoneal abscess can arise secondary to pancreatitis, spinal infection, retroperitoneal perforation of peptic ulcer, interventions such as ERCP, or upper renal tract infections. Plain film diagnosis requires a high degree of vigilance. CT or ultrasound examinations are the preferred methods of investigation of intra-abdominal collections.

CASE 8.6

Age: 38 years	Gender: Male
Clinical problem: Chronic cough and sputum production	
Images in exam case: Plain radiograph (1), CT (5)	

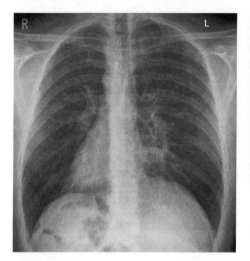

Figure 48a

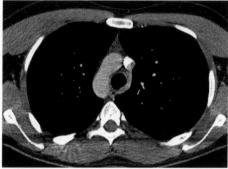

Figure 48b

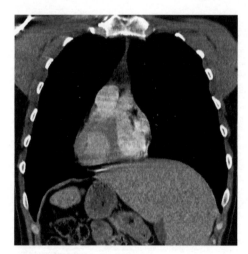

Figure 48c

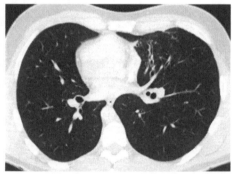

Figure 48d

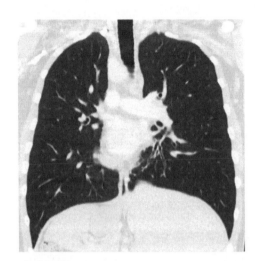

Figure 48e

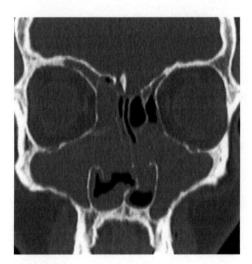

Figure 48f

FINDINGS

1. Chest X-ray:
    a. Dextrocardia
    b. No gastric bubble visualised on the left upper quadrant.
2. CT thorax:
    a. Right-sided aortic arch and SVC on the left side
    b. Cardiac apex on the right side
    c. Liver on the left and spleen on the right side
    d. Cylindrical dilatation of the bronchi of the left middle lobe
    e. Extensive opacification of bilateral paranasal sinuses, with bilateral widening of the osteomeatal complex.

INTERPRETATION

Situs inversus, bronchiectasis of the left middle lobe and sinonasal polyposis.

DIAGNOSIS

Kartagener syndrome.

FURTHER INVESTIGATIONS AND MANAGEMENT

1. If the patient is infertile, sperm motility studies may be necessary.
2. Respiratory and ENT referral for management of bronchiectasis and sinus mucosal disease.

FURTHER INFORMATION

Kartagener syndrome is a primary ciliary dyskinesia syndrome – a combination of bronchiectasis, nasal polyposis with sinusitis and situs inversus. In males it can be associated with immotile spermatozoa and consequent infertility. It is an autosomal recessive genetic abnormality. Approximately 20% of patients with situs inversus have Kartagener syndrome, whereas 50% of patients with immotile cilia syndrome have situs inversus and the remaining 50% have situs solitus.

Chapter 2
Rapid reporting

Abdomen

Figures AXR1 to AXR9

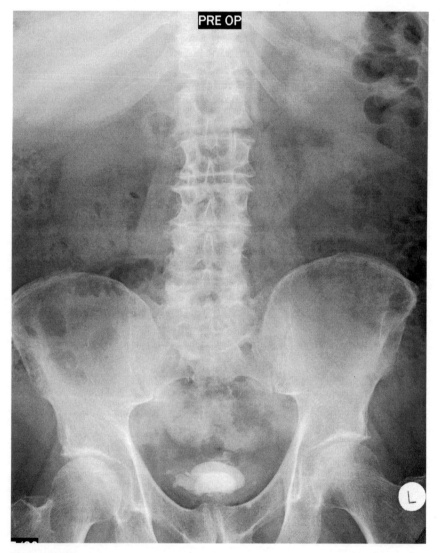

Figure AXR1

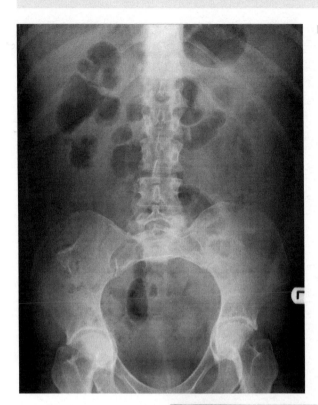

Figure AXR2

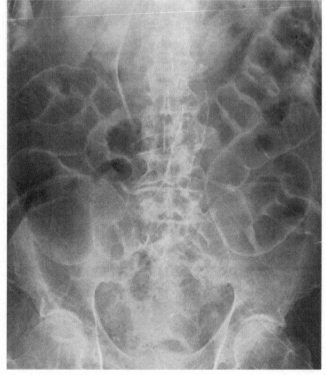

Figure AXR3

Figure AXR4

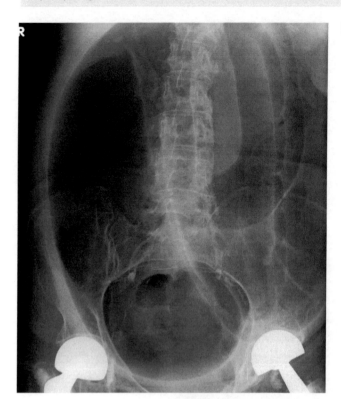

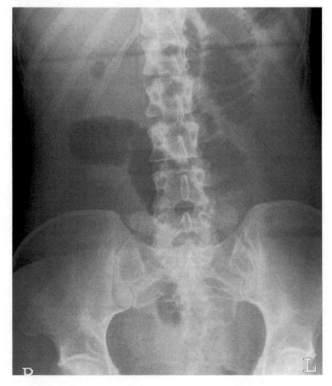

Figure AXR5

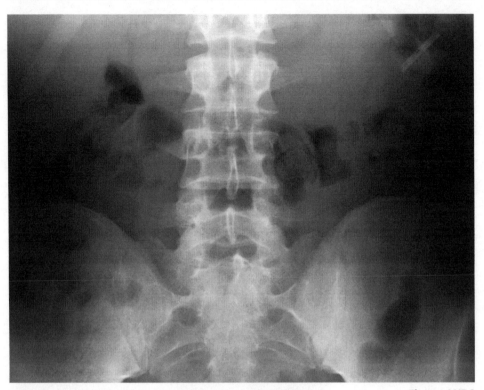

Figure AXR6

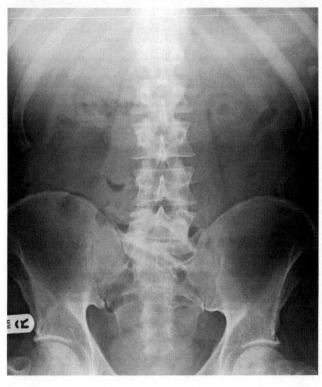

Figure AXR7

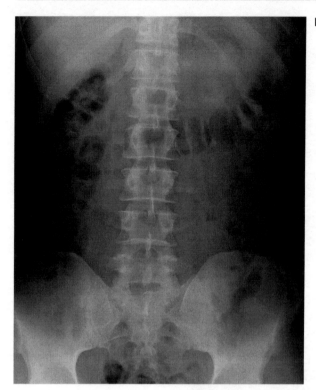

Figure AXR8

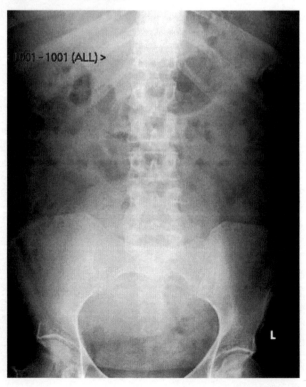

1001 – 1001 (ALL) >

L

Figure AXR9

ANSWERS: ABDOMEN

AXR1 – Bladder calculi
AXR2 – Iliac wings (Fong's syndrome)
AXR3 – Pneumoperitoneum
AXR4 – Sigmoid volvulus
AXR5 – Small bowel obstruction (small bowel dilatation)
AXR6 – Swallowed foreign body (razor)
AXR7 – Thumb printing of transverse colon (colitis)
AXR8 – Left 12th rib destruction
AXR9 – Pelvic mass

Chest

Figures CXR1 to CXR21

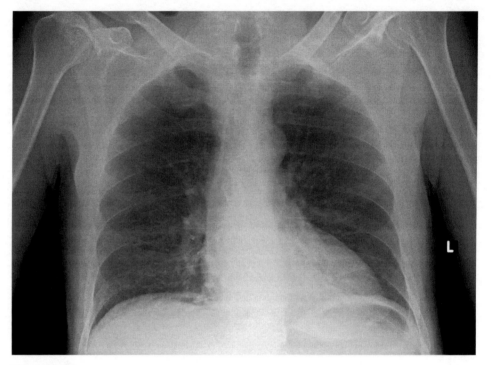

Figure CXR1

Figure CXR2

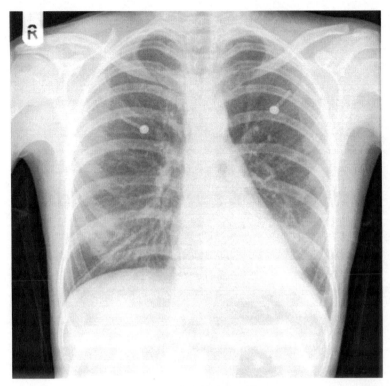

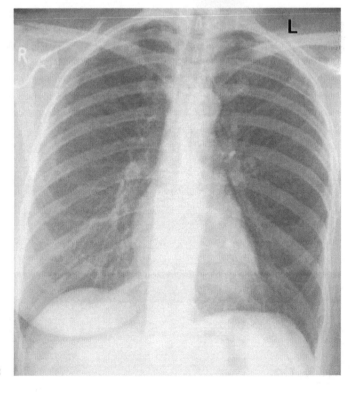

Figure CXR3

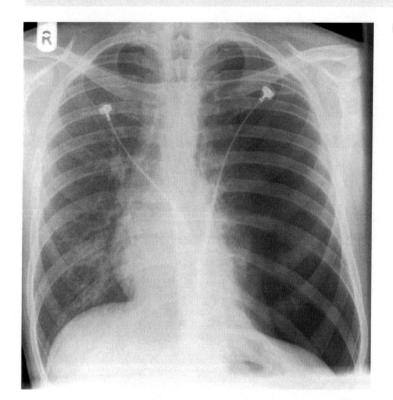

Figure CXR4

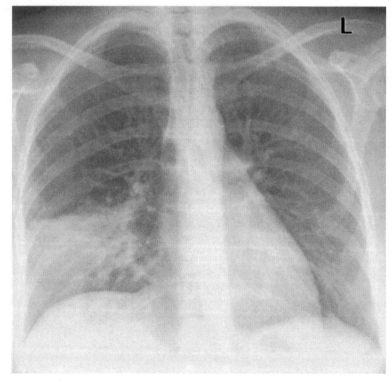

Figure CXR5

Figure CXR6

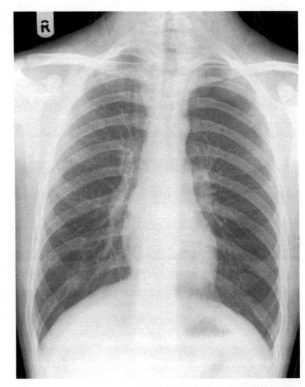

Figure CXR7

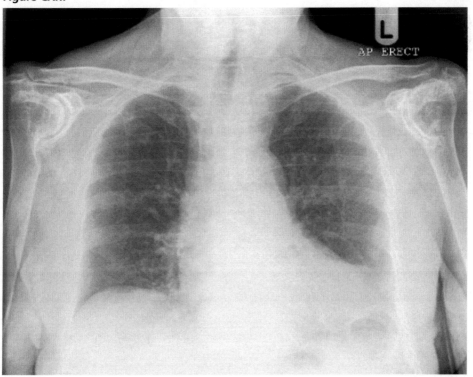

Figure CXR8

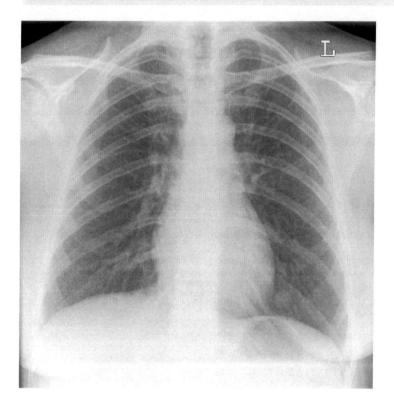

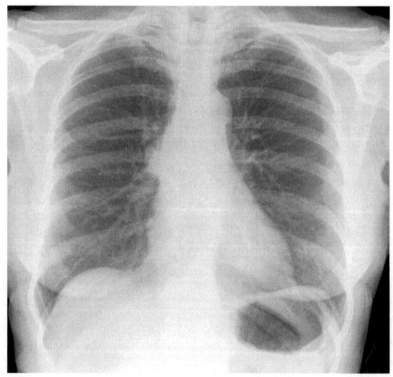

Figure CXR9

Figure CXR10

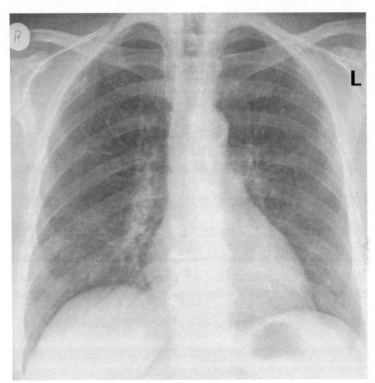

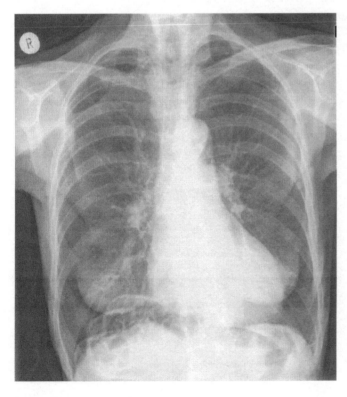

Figure CXR11

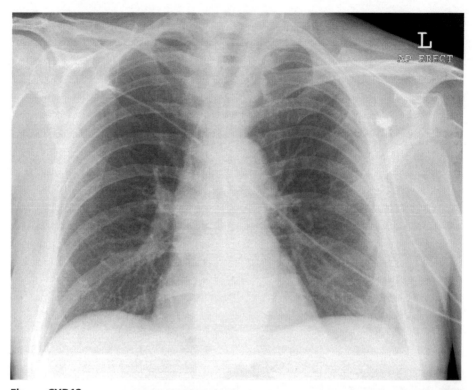

Figure CXR12

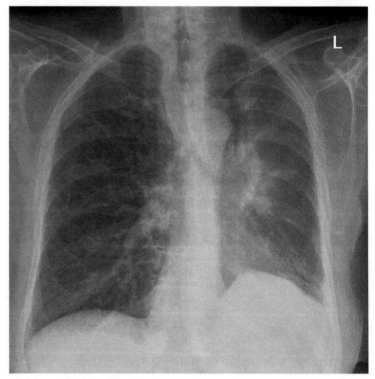

Figure CXR13

Figure CXR14

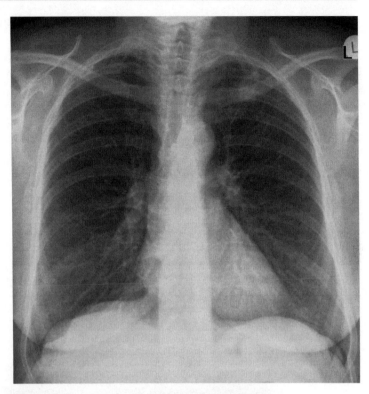

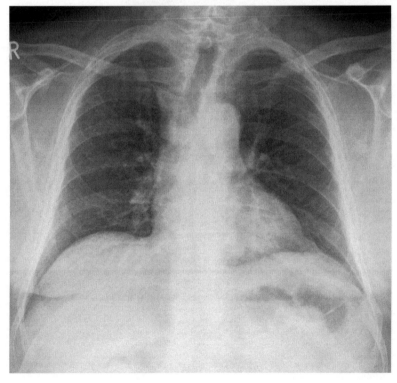

Figure CXR15

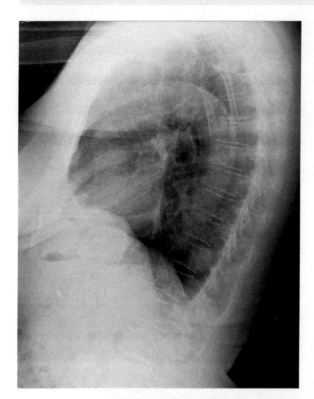

Figure CXR16

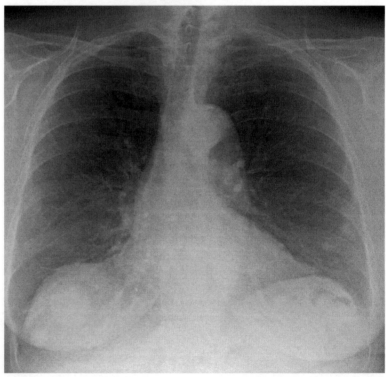

Figure CXR17

Figure CXR18

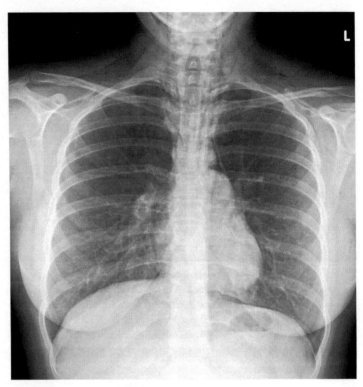

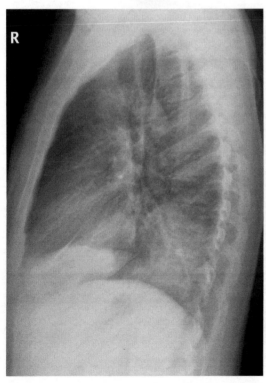

Figure CXR19

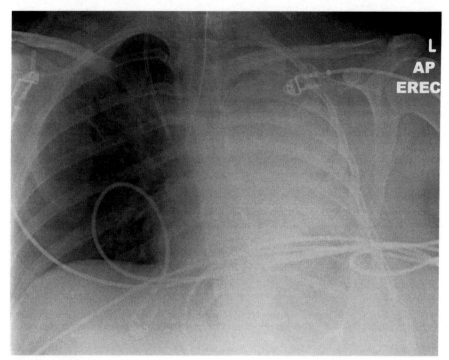

Figure CXR20

Figure CXR21

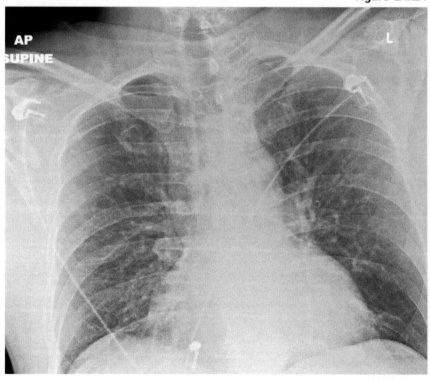

ANSWERS: CHEST

CXR1 – Pneumoperitoneum
CXR2 – Left lower lobe collapse
CXR3 – Left mastectomy
CXR4 – Left tension pneumothorax
CXR5 – Right middle lobe consolidation
CXR6 – Left pneumothorax
CXR7 – Rheumatoid arthritis of both shoulder joints
CXR8 – Left lower lobe nodule
CXR9 – Right hilar mass
CXR10 – Left 5th and 6th rib fractures
CXR11 – Right 4th rib destructive lesion
CXR12 – Fracture dislocation of left humeral head
CXR13 – Left upper lobe collapse
CXR14 – Left apical mass
CXR15 – Left scapula destructive lesion (metastasis)
CXR16 – Lung base mass
CXR17 – Multiple lung metastases
CXR18 – Pneumomediastinum
CXR19 – Right lower lobe consolidation
CXR20 – Right main bronchus intubation
CXR21 – Right scapula fracture

Skull

Figures SXR1 to SXR5

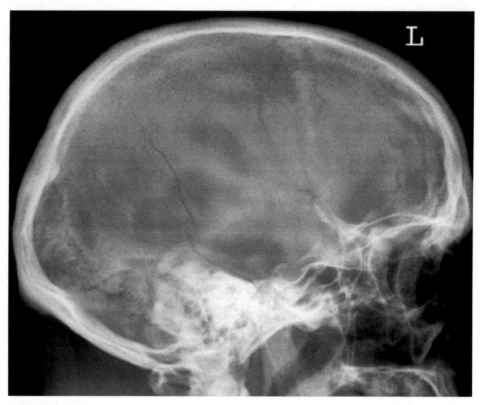

Figure SXR1

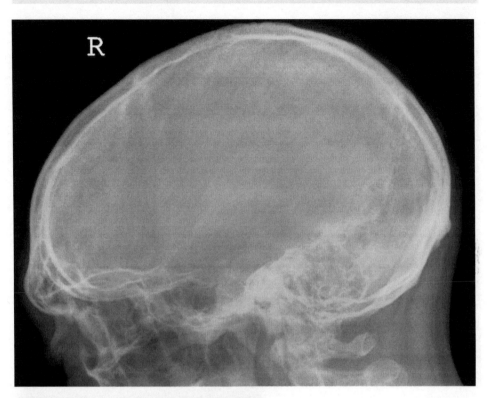

Figure SXR2

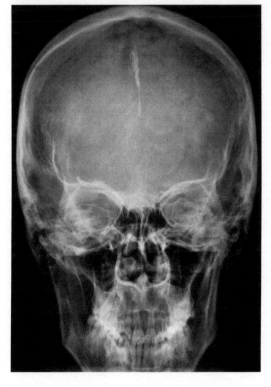

Figure SXR3

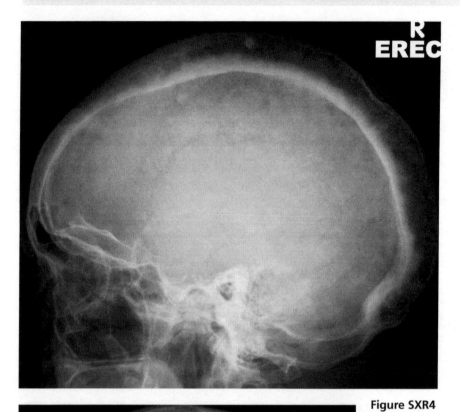

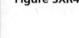

Figure SXR4

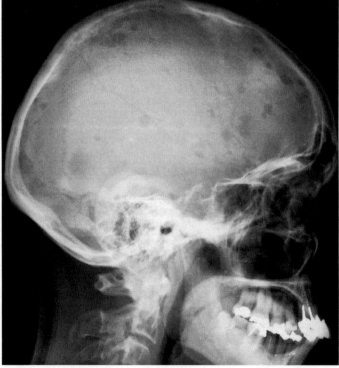

Figure SXR5

ANSWERS: SKULL

SXR1 – Fractured temporal bone
SXR2 – Air-fluid level sphenoid sinus
SXR3 – Cystic lesion right mandible
SXR4 – Paget's disease (skull vault thickening)
SXR5 – Multiple myeloma (multiple lytic lesions)

Facial bones

Figures FAC1 to FAC6

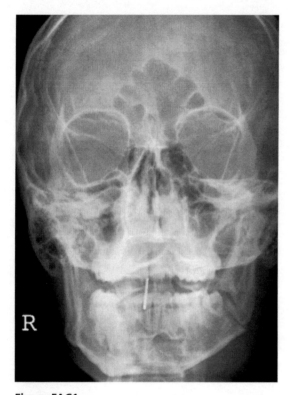

Figure FAC1

Figure FAC2

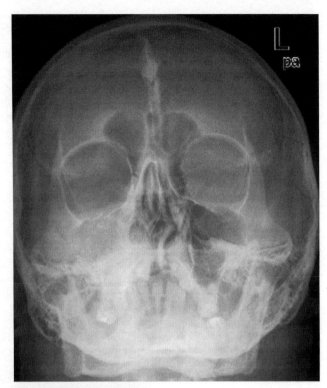

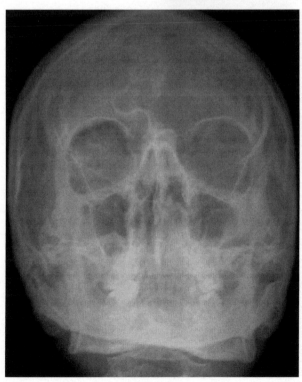

Figure FAC3

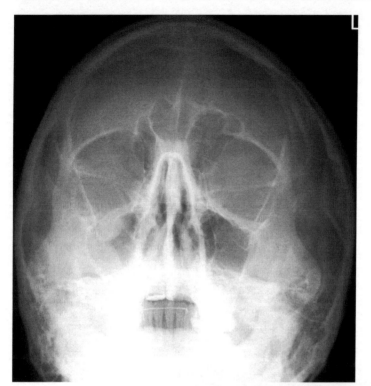

Figure FAC4

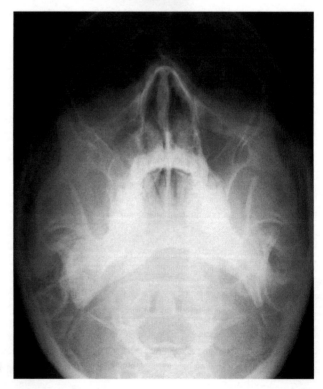

Figure FAC5

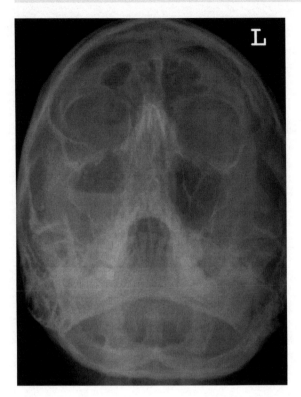

Figure FAC6

ANSWERS: FACIAL BONES

FAC1 – Fractured left angle of mandible
FAC2 – Opacification of right maxillary antrum
FAC3 – Right orbital emphysema
FAC4 – Right orbital floor fracture
FAC5 – Right tripod fracture
FAC6 – Air-fluid level in right maxillary antrum

Cervical spine

Figures CSP1 to CSP12

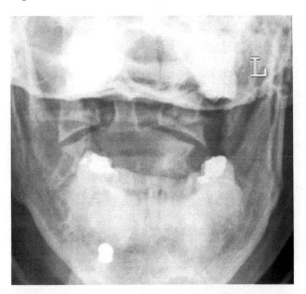

Figure CSP1

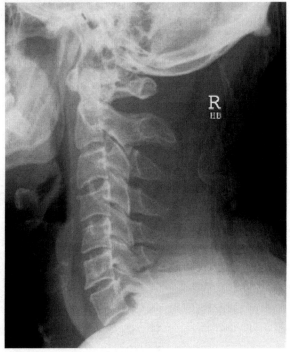

Figure CSP2

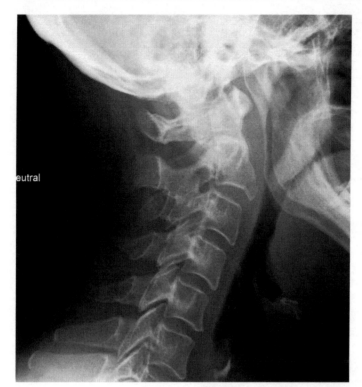

Figure CSP3

eutral

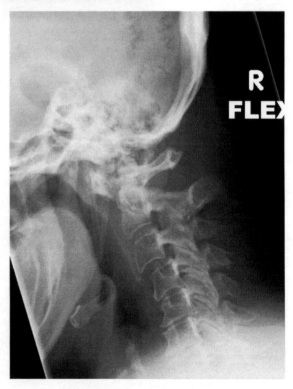

Figure CSP4

Figure CSP5

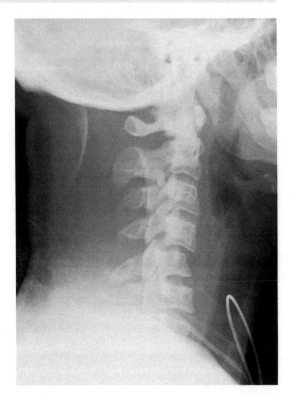

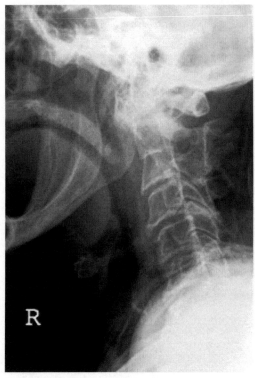

Figure CSP6

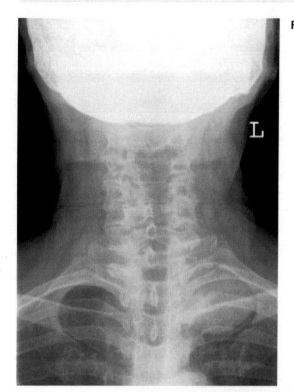

Figure CSP7

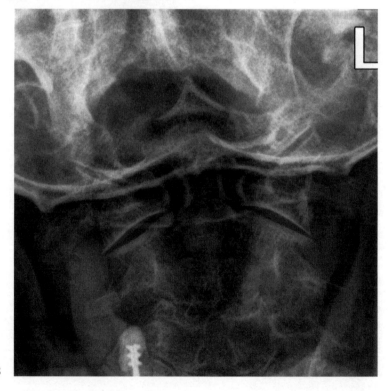

Figure CSP8

Figure CSP9

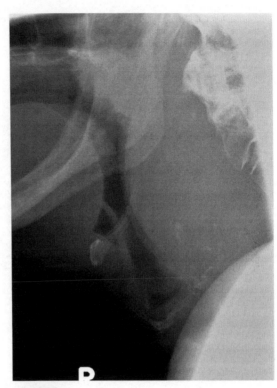

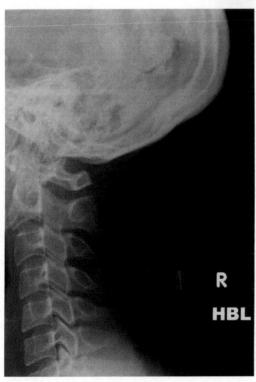

Figure CSP10

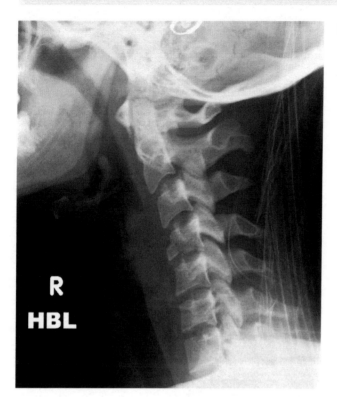

Figure CSP11

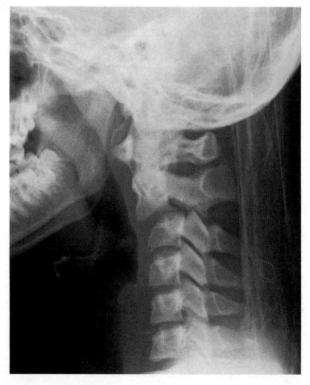

Figure CSP12

ANSWERS: CERVICAL SPINE

CSP1 – Fractured C1
CSP2 – Fractured C6 spinous process
CSP3 – Fractured C2 anteroinferior corner
CSP4 – Atlanto-axial subluxation
CSP5 – C4–5 unifacet dislocation
CSP6 – Fractured C2 vertebral body
CSP7 – Left apical mass
CSP8 – Type II odontoid peg fracture
CSP9 – Prevertebral soft tissue swelling
CSP10 – Fractured skull
CSP11 – Flexion teardrop fracture of C4 vertebral body
CSP12 – Perched facet C2 on C3

Thoracic spine

Figures TS1 to TS2

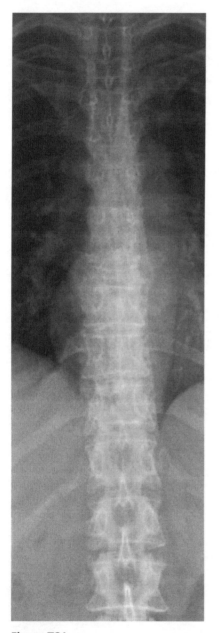

Figure TS1

Figure TS2

ANSWERS: THORACIC SPINE

TS1 – Fractured T8 with paraspinal swelling
TS2 – Right-sided lung mass

Lumbosacral spine

Figures LS1 to LS6

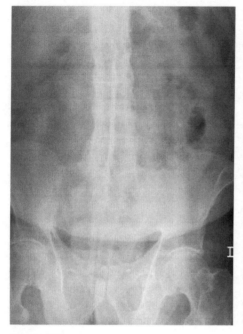

Figure LS1

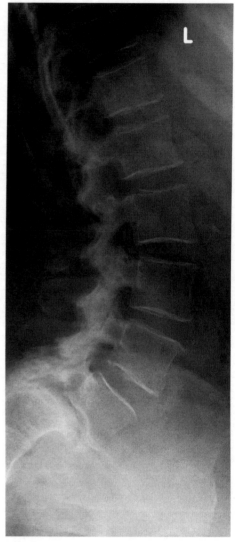

Figure LS2

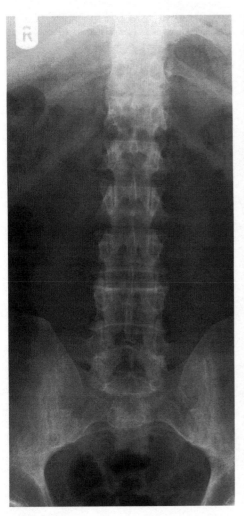

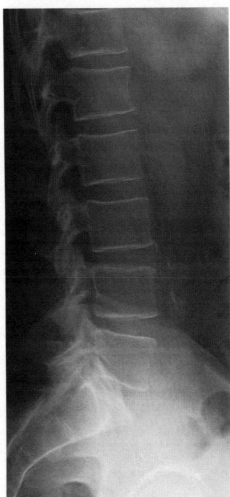

Figure LS3   **Figure LS4**

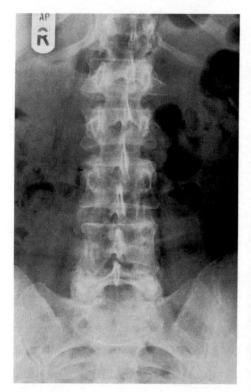

Figure LS5

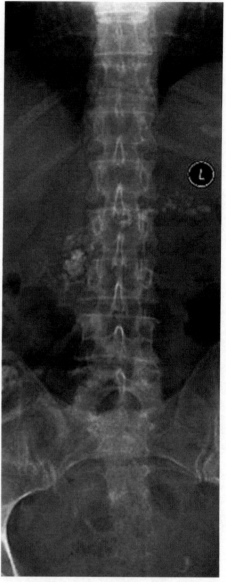

Figure LS6

ANSWERS: LUMBOSACRAL SPINE

LS1 – Ankylosing spondylitis
LS2 – L5–S1 anterolisthesis
LS3 – Bilateral sacroiliitis
LS4 – Lytic lesion of T12 vertebral body
LS5 – Lytic lesion of right L4 pedicle
LS6 – Pancreatic calcification

Shoulder

Figures SH1 to SH14

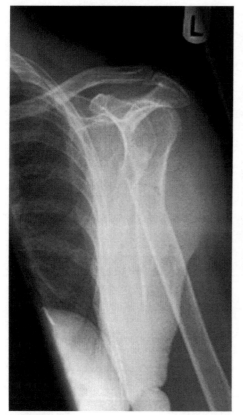

Figure SH1

Figure SH2

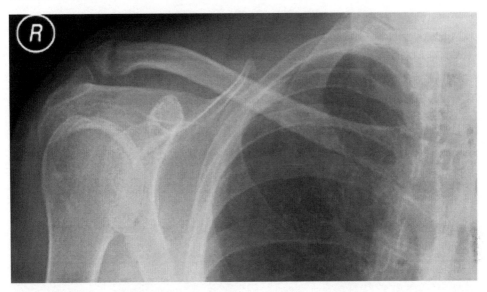

Figure SH3

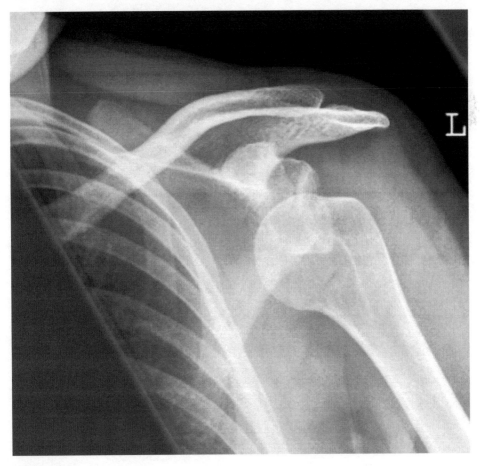

Figure SH4

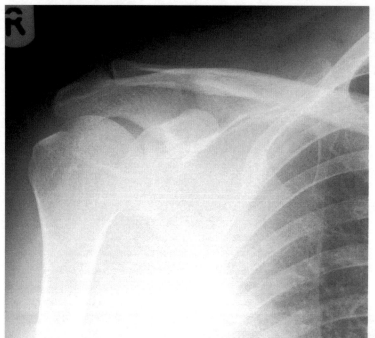

Figure SH5

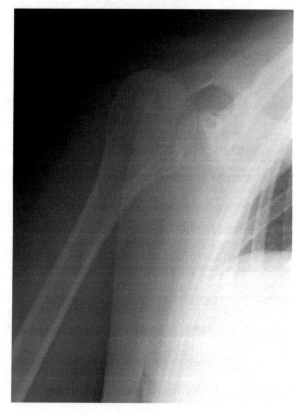

Figure SH6

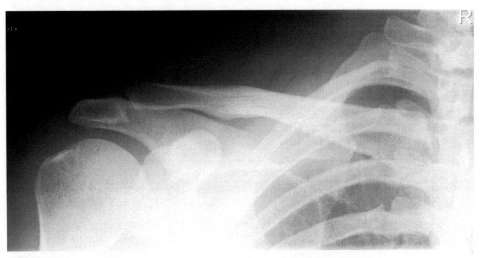

Figure SH7

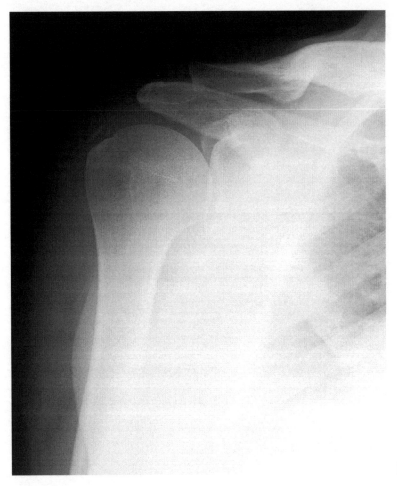

Figure SH8

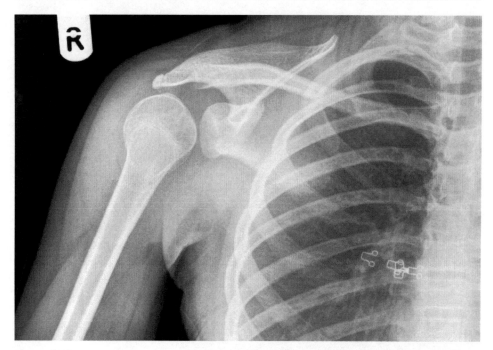

Figure SH9

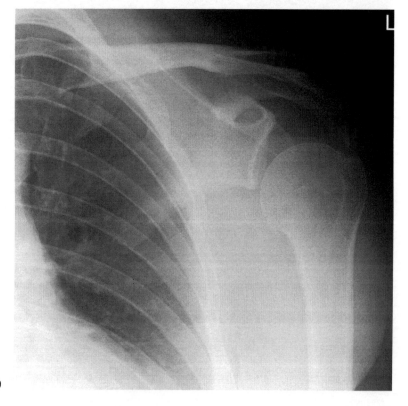

Figure SH10

Figure SH11

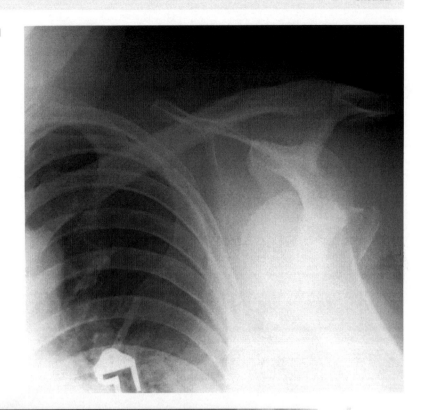

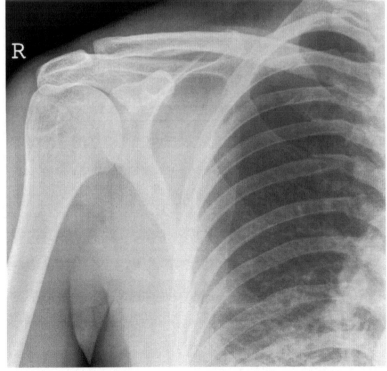

Figure SH12

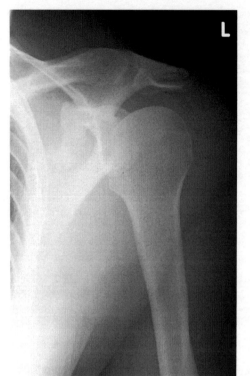

Figure SH13

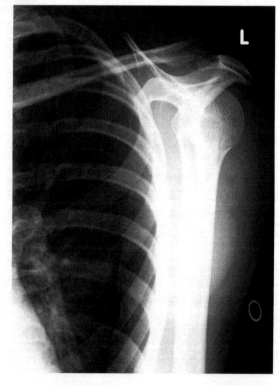

Figure SH14

ANSWERS: SHOULDER

SH1 – Fractured shaft of left humerus
SH2 – Anterior dislocation of humeral head
SH3 – Fractured distal clavicle
SH4 – Anterior dislocation of humeral head
SH5 – Fractured scapula
SH6 – Posterior dislocation of humeral head
SH7 – Acromioclavicular joint disruption
SH8 – Calcific tendonitis
SH9 – Posterior dislocation of humeral head
SH10 – Fractured greater tuberosity and lipohaemarthrosis
SH11 – Hill–Sachs fracture dislocation
SH12 – Pneumothorax
SH13 – Fractured acromion
SH14 – Posterior dislocation of humeral head

Elbow

Figures ELB1 to ELB12

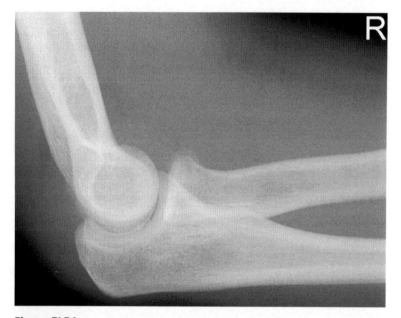

Figure ELB1

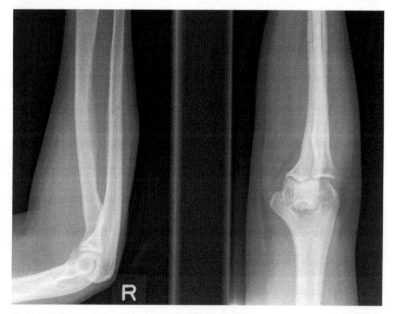

Figure ELB2

Figure ELB3

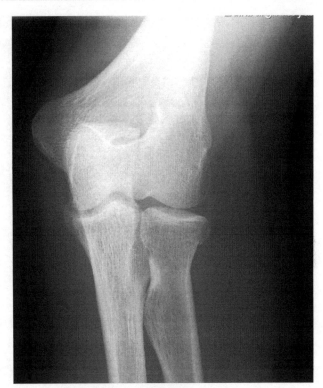

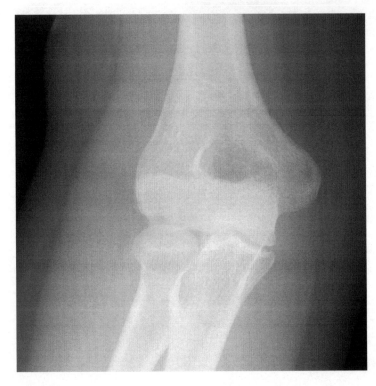

Figure ELB4

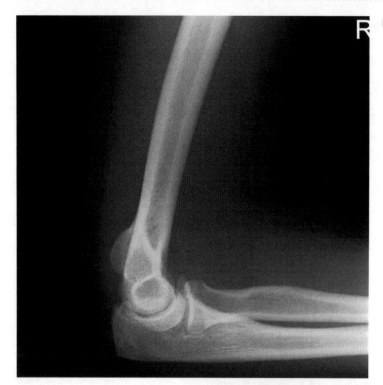

Figure ELB5

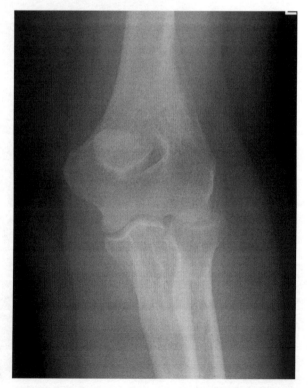

Figure ELB6

Figure ELB7

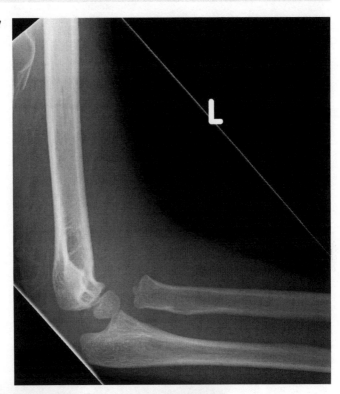

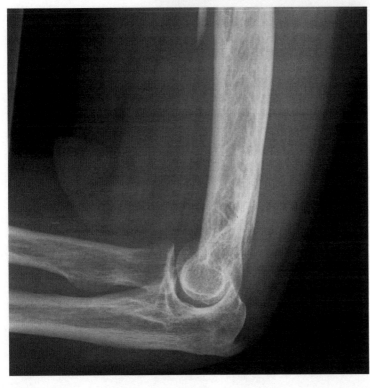

Figure ELB8

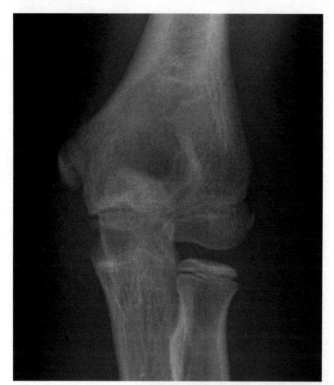

Figure ELB9

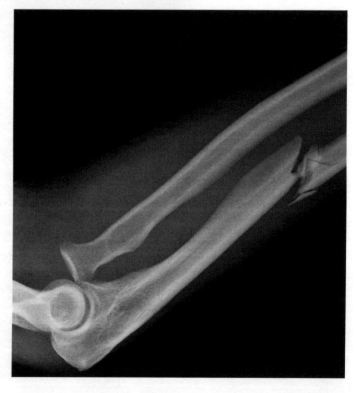

Figure ELB10

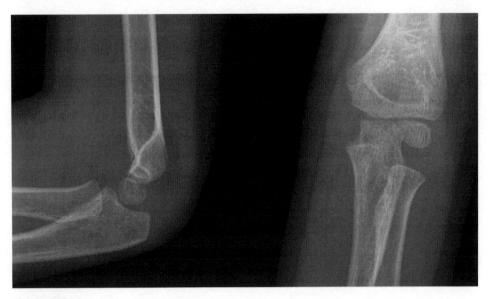

Figure ELB11

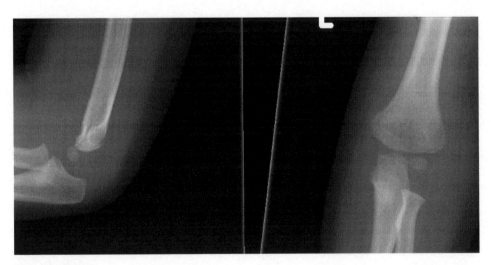

Figure ELB12

ANSWERS: ELBOW

ELB1 – Fractured radius
ELB2 – Fractured midshaft ulna
ELB3 – Fractured radial neck
ELB4 – Fractured capitellum
ELB5 – Fractured coronoid process
ELB6 – Fractured olecranon process
ELB7 – Radial head dislocation
ELB8 – Fractured humerus
ELB9 – Lateral epicondyle avulsion fracture
ELB10 – Monteggia fracture dislocation
ELB11 – Supracondylar fracture
ELB12 – Lateral condylar fracture

Wrist

Figures WR1 to WR7

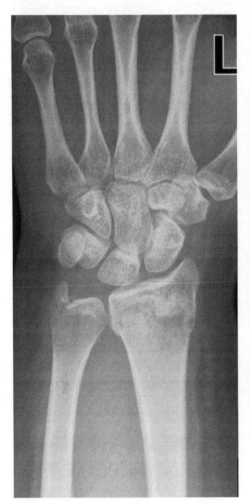

Figure WR1

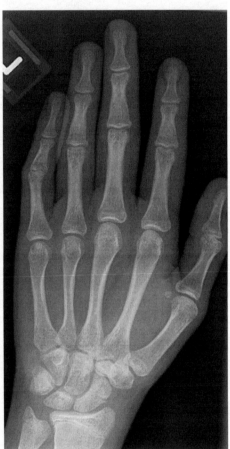

Figure WR2

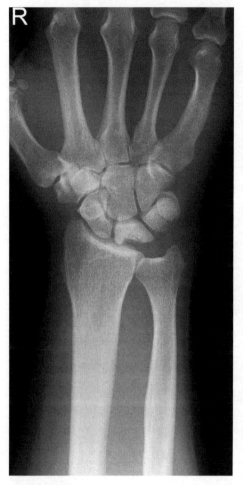

Figure WR3

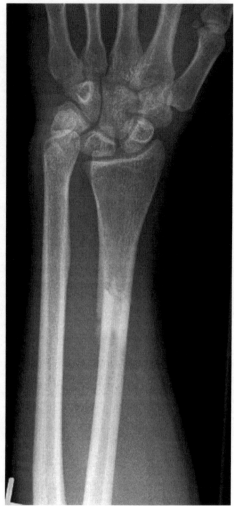

Figure WR4

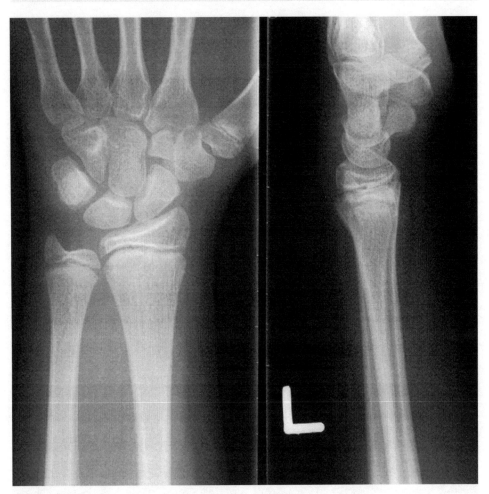

Figure WR5

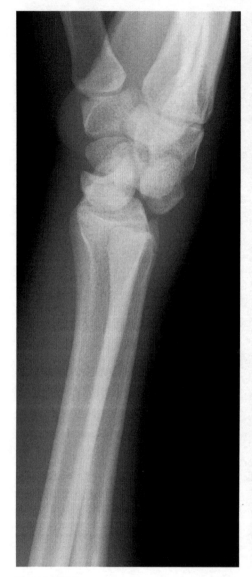

Figure WR6

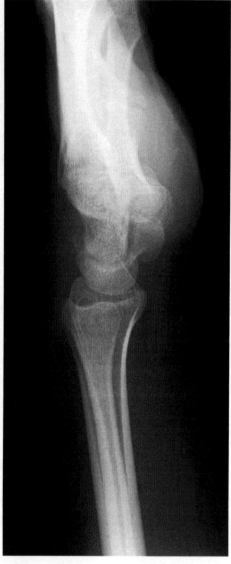

Figure WR7

ANSWERS: WRIST

WR1 – Fractured distal radius
WR2 – Fractured scaphoid
WR3 – Kienbock's disease
WR4 – Galeazzi fracture dislocation
WR5 – Fractured distal radius
WR6 – Perilunate dislocation
WR7 – Fractured triquetrum

Hand

Figures HAN1 to HAN13

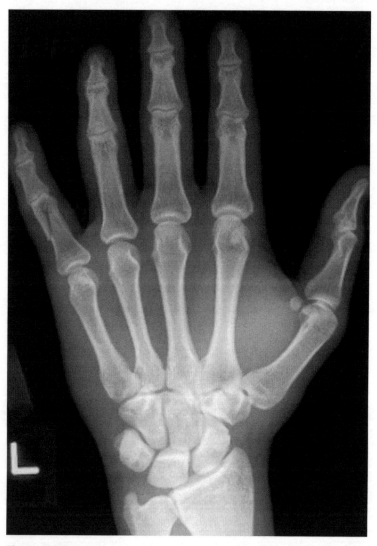

Figure HAN1

Figure HAN2

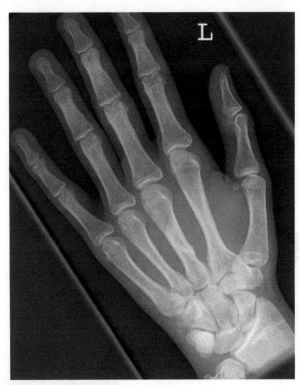

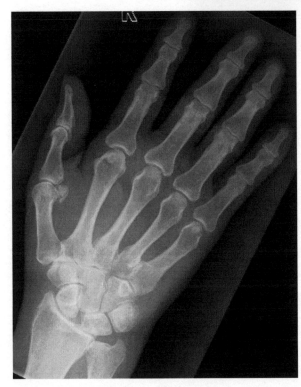

Figure HAN3

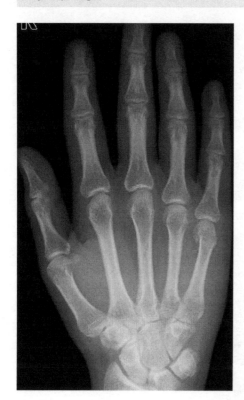

Figure HAN4

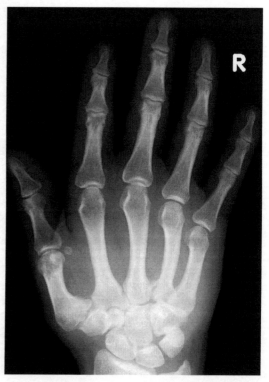

Figure HAN5

Figure HAN6

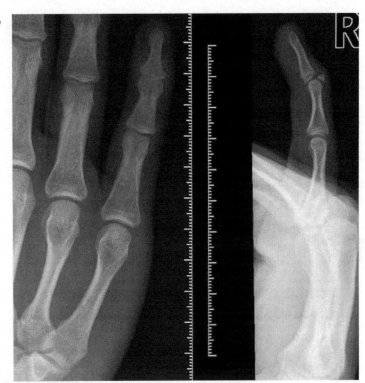

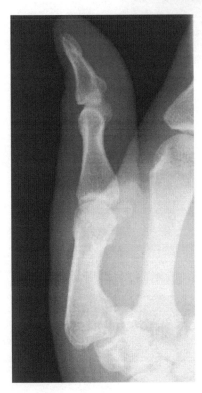

Figure HAN7

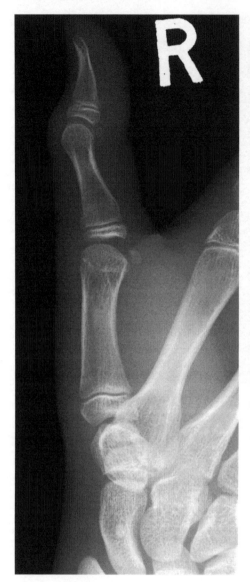

Figure HAN8

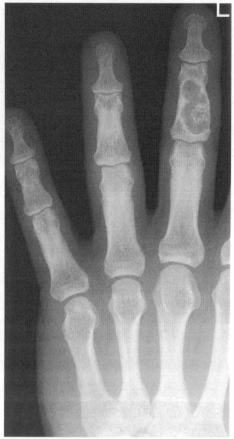

Figure HAN9

Figure HAN10

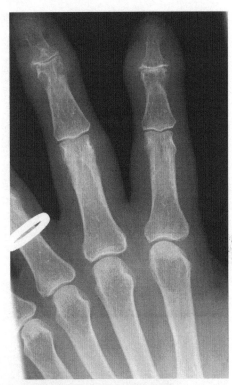

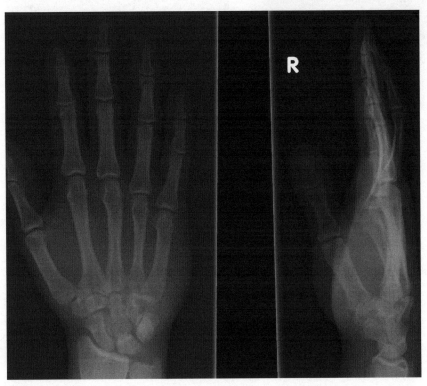

Figure HAN11

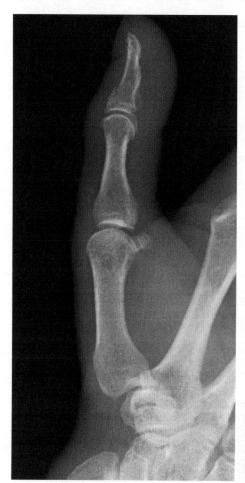

Figure HAN12

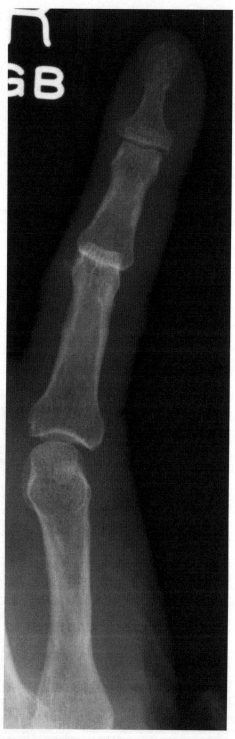

Figure HAN13

ANSWERS: HAND

HAN1 – Fractured proximal phalanx of little finger
HAN2 – Fractured shaft of 3rd metacarpal
HAN3 – Scapholunate dissociation
HAN4 – Fractured neck of 5th metacarpal
HAN5 – Dislocated base of 4th and 5th metacarpals
HAN6 – Fractured base of distal phalanx of little finger
HAN7 – Bennett's fracture
HAN8 – Fractured proximal phalanx of thumb
HAN9 – Enchondroma
HAN10 – Gout (erosions)
HAN11 – Fractured hamate
HAN12 – Fractured distal phalanx of thumb
HAN13 – Dislocated proximal interphalangeal joint of little finger

Pelvis

Figures PEL1 to PEL10

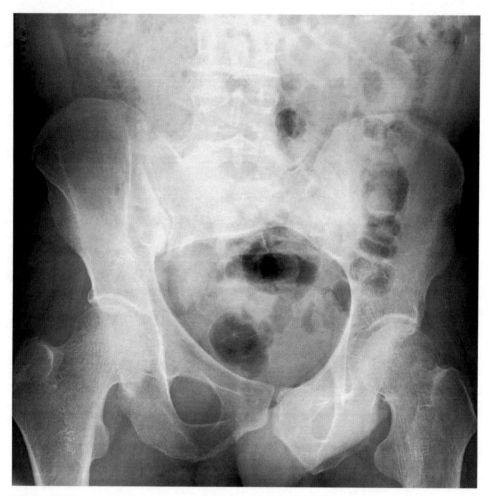

Figure PEL1

Figure PEL2

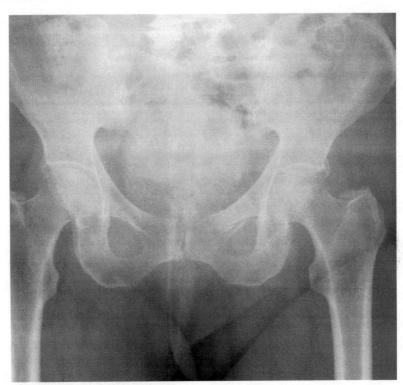

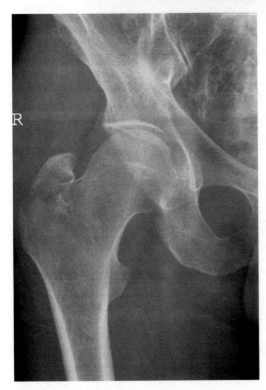

Figure PEL3

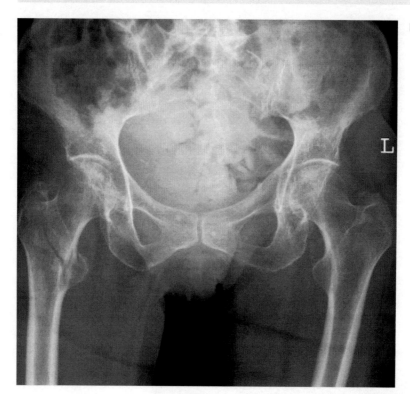

Figure PEL4

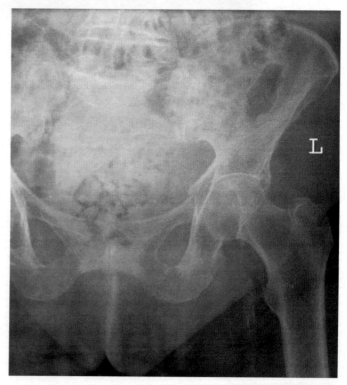

Figure PEL5

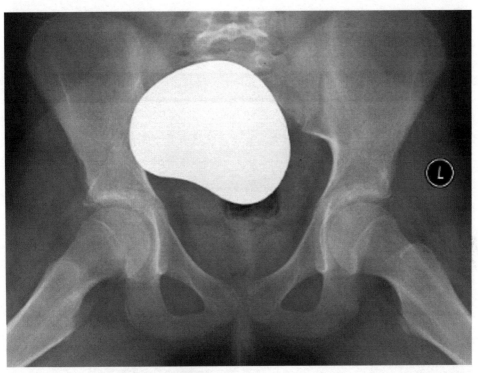

Figure PEL6

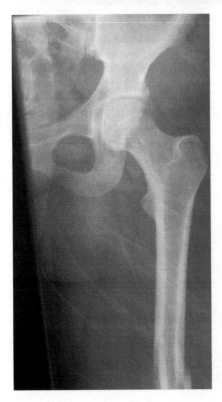

Figure PEL7

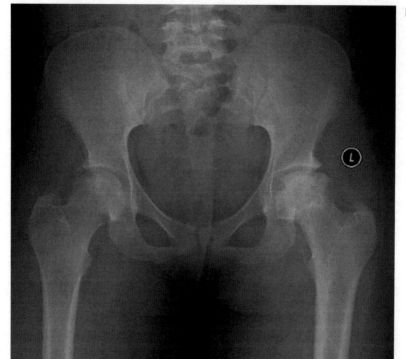

Figure PEL8

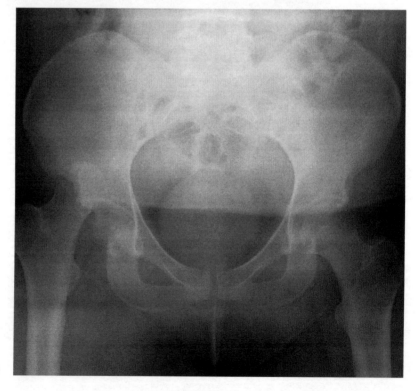

Figure PEL9

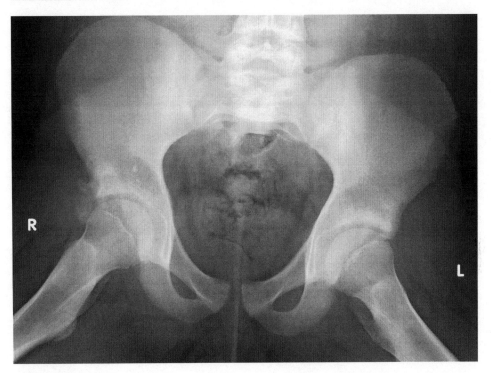

Figure PEL10

ANSWERS: PELVIS

PEL1 – Fractured left neck of femur

PEL2 – Fractured left superior pubic ramus

PEL3 – Fractured right greater trochanter

PEL4 – Intertrochanteric fracture of right femur

PEL5 – Fractured left acetabulum

PEL6 – Right slipped upper femoral epiphysis

PEL7 – Fractured left femoral shaft

PEL8 – Avascular necrosis of left femoral head

PEL9 – Right femoral head dislocation

PEL10 – Avulsion fracture of right anterior inferior iliac spine

Knee

Figures KN1 to KN10

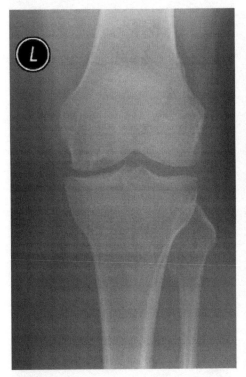

Figure KN1

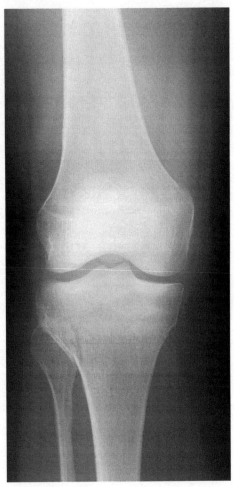

Figure KN2

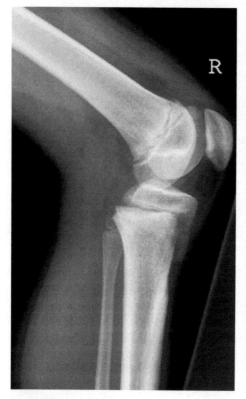

Figure KN3

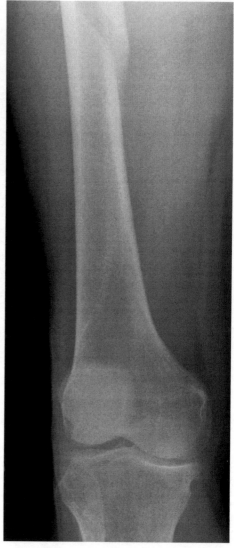

Figure KN4

Figure KN5

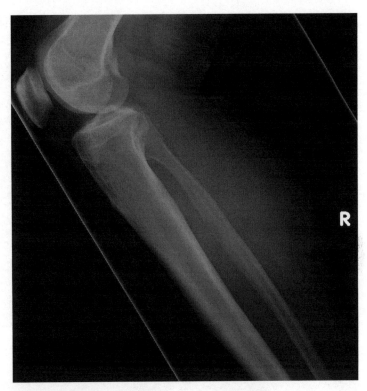

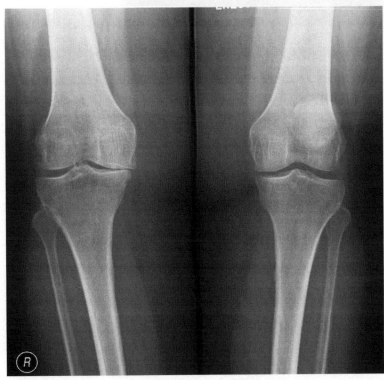

Figure KN6

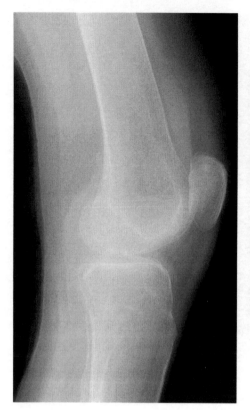

Figure KN7

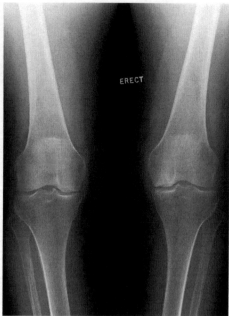

Figure KN8

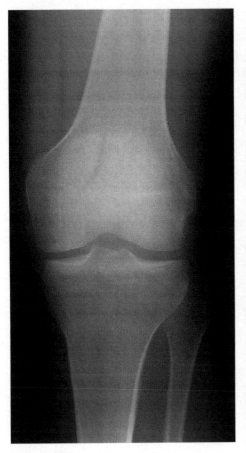

Figure KN9

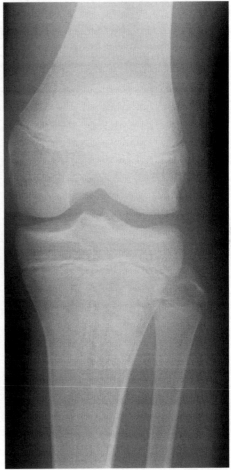

Figure KN10

ANSWERS: KNEE

KN1 – Osteochondral damage to medial femoral condyle
KN2 – Fractured lateral tibial plateau
KN3 – Salter–Harris type II fracture of proximal tibia
KN4 – Fractured femoral shaft
KN5 – Fractured neck of fibula
KN6 – Absent right patella
KN7 – Lipohaemarthrosis
KN8 – Osteochondritis dissecans of the bilateral medial femoral condyles
KN9 – Fractured patella
KN10 – Segond fracture

Ankle

Figures ANK1 to ANK10

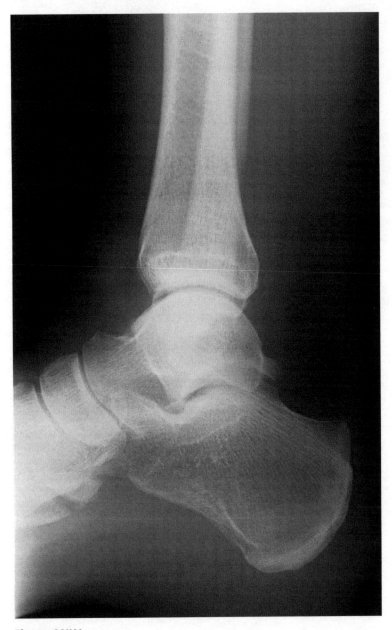

Figure ANK1

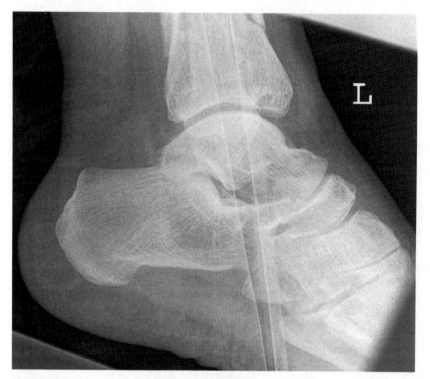

Figure ANK2

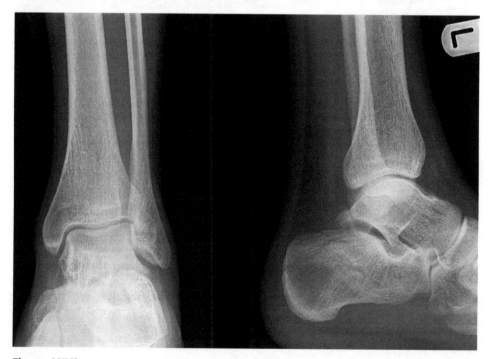

Figure ANK3

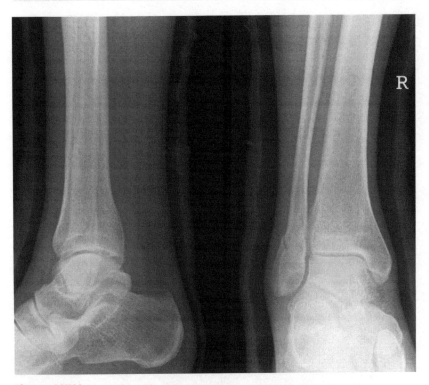

Figure ANK4

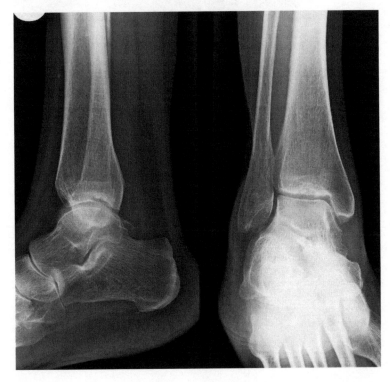

Figure ANK5

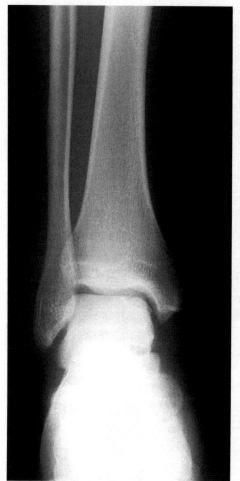

Figure ANK6

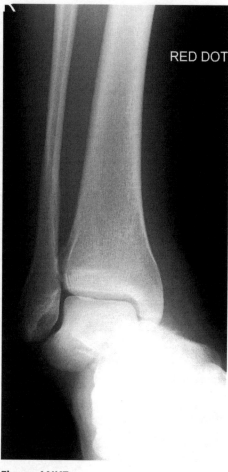

RED DOT

Figure ANK7

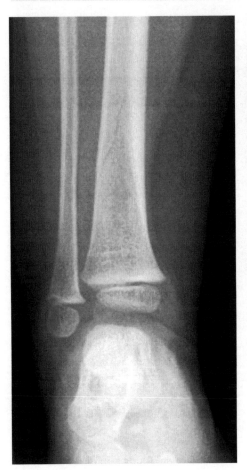

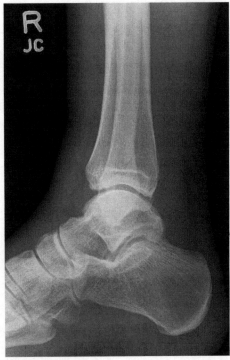

Figure ANK9

Figure ANK8

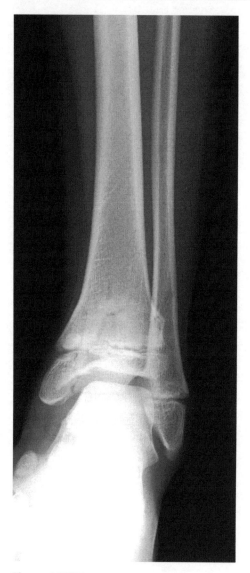

Figure ANK10

ANSWERS: ANKLE

ANK1 – Fractured base of 5th metatarsal
ANK2 – Fractured distal tibia
ANK3 – Fractured calcaneum
ANK4 – Fractured distal fibula
ANK5 – Osteochondral damage to distal tibia
ANK6 – Osteochondral damage to talar dome
ANK7 – Fractured talus
ANK8 – Toddler's fracture
ANK9 – Fractured distal fibula
ANK10 – Salter–Harris type IV fracture of distal tibia

Foot

Figures FT1 to FT10

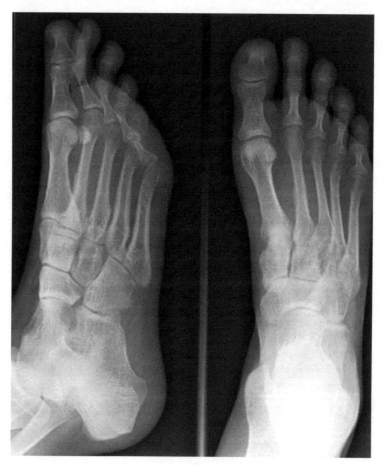

Figure FT1

Figure FT2

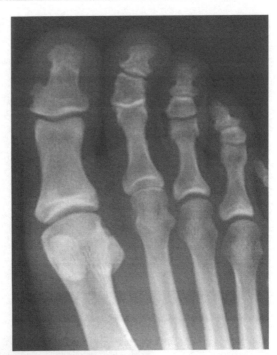

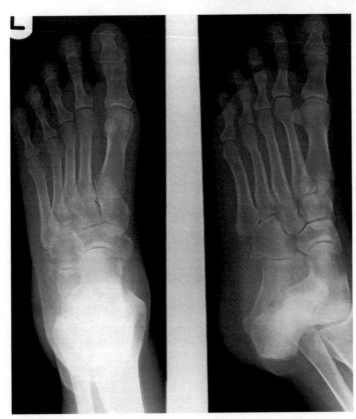

Figure FT3

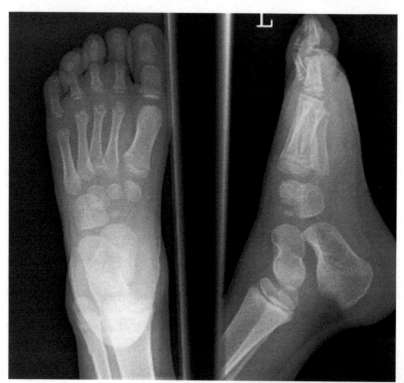

Figure FT4

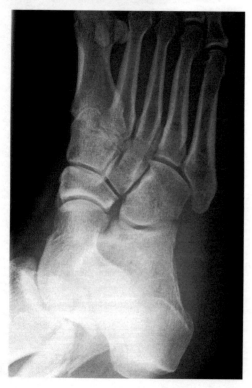

Figure FT5

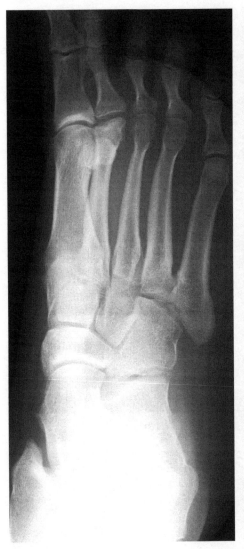

Figure FT6

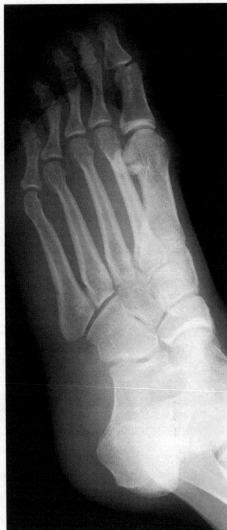

Figure FT7

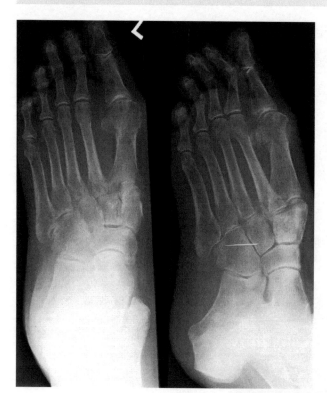

Figure FT8

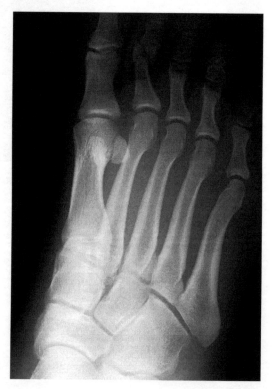

Figure FT9

Figure FT10

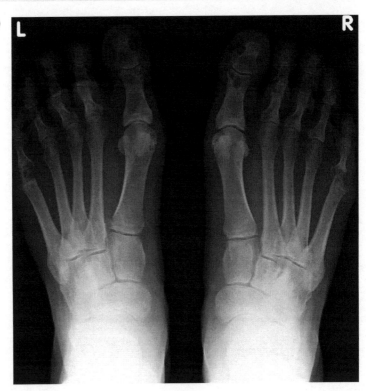

ANSWERS: FOOT

FT1 – Stress fracture of 2nd metatarsal

FT2 – Dislocated proximal interphalangeal joint of 2nd toe

FT3 – Fractured base of 5th metatarsal

FT4 – Fractured distal fibula

FT5 – Fractured distal fibula

FT6 – Frieberg's disease

FT7 – Jones fracture

FT8 – Lisfranc dislocation

FT9 – Fractured proximal phalanx of 2nd toe

FT10 – Rheumatoid arthritis (erosive arthritis)

Chapter 3
Oral examinations

Viva 1

CASE 1.1: 66-YEAR-OLD MAN WITH ACUTE LOWER ABDOMINAL PAIN AND RECTAL BLEEDING

Figure v1.1a

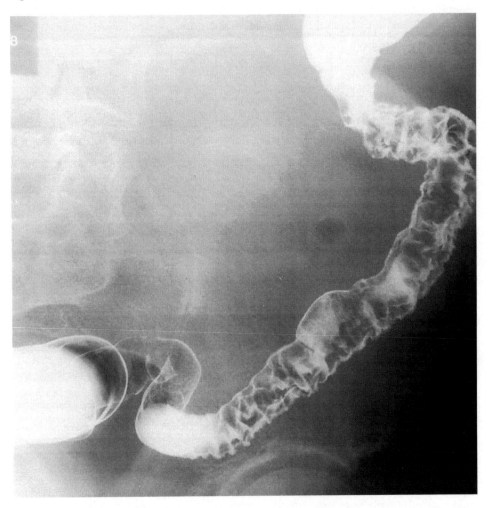

ACUTE ISCHAEMIC COLITIS

FINDINGS

Double-contrast barium enema examination, oblique projection:
1. Long segment mucosal thickening and irregularity of the sigmoid colon
2. Loss of haustral markings
3. 'Thumb printing.'

MAIN DIAGNOSIS

Appearance consistent with colitis. In view of the distribution of colitis in the watershed area of arterial supply and marked 'thumb printing', the most likely aetiology is ischaemic colitis.

DIFFERENTIAL DIAGNOSIS

1. Infective colitis (e.g. pseudomembranous colitis). There would be a history of antibiotic use prior to development of colitis.
2. Ulcerative colitis. However, this is unlikely as the distal colon appears normal, although patients on therapeutic enemas may have rectal sparing.
3. Crohn's colitis. However, there is no evidence of aphthoid or deep ulcers, or pseudodiverticula.

FURTHER INVESTIGATIONS AND MANAGEMENT

1. As arterial thromboembolism is a cause of ischaemic colitis, check the ECG for atrial fibrillation and explore risk factors for atherosclerosis.
2. A minority of patients may develop gangrene and perforation, so watch for signs of peritonitis.
3. CT abdomen/CT mesenteric angiography may or may not be necessary.

FURTHER INFORMATION

Ischaemic colitis is most commonly due to small vessel disease. Arterial thromboembolism and venous thrombosis are less common causes of ischaemic colitis. Splenic flexure is the watershed region between the SMA and IMA distribution, and rectosigmoid colon is the watershed region between IMA and inferior hypogastric artery distribution. Both regions are vulnerable to ischaemic insult. Bowel infarction and perforation are serious complications of ischaemic colitis. Pneumatosis is a sign of gangrenous bowel wall. Transmural bowel infarction can give rise to fibrosis and ischaemic stricture.

CASE 1.2: 45-YEAR-OLD MAN WITH DIARRHOEA

Figure v1.2a

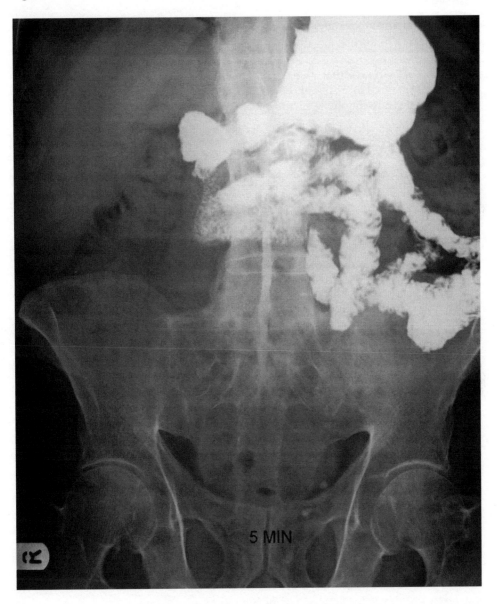

5 MIN

ANKYLOSING SPONDYLITIS

FINDINGS

Barium follow-through study, 5-minute post-contrast film:
1. D-J flexure in normal anatomical position
2. No mucosal abnormality of the proximal small bowel
3. Fusion of both sacroiliac joints
4. Densely ossified interspinous ligament giving a thick vertical line ('dagger sign')
5. Marginal syndesmophytes giving a 'bamboo' spine appearance.

MAIN DIAGNOSIS

1. Ankylosing spondylitis.
2. Normal proximal small bowel mucosa.

DIFFERENTIAL DIAGNOSIS

1. Arthropathy associated with inflammatory bowel disease. The skeletal features are very similar to those of ankylosing spondylitis.
2. Psoriatic arthritis. However, syndesmophytes are usually large, bulky and non-marginal.
3. Reiter's syndrome. However, sacroiliitis is usually bilateral and asymmetrical.

FURTHER INVESTIGATIONS AND MANAGEMENT

1. Assessment of the whole of the small bowel, including the terminal ileum.
2. Review previous radiographs.
3. HLA-B27.
4. Colonoscopy and biopsy to look for evidence of inflammatory bowel disease.

FURTHER INFORMATION

In any abdominal radiograph the visualised skeleton must be assessed carefully. Other classic exam cases are colonic mucosal thickening with sacroiliitis, gallstones, or avascular necrosis of head of femur.

HLA-B27 spondyloarthropathies are as follows:
1. ankylosing spondylitis (bilateral and symmetrical sacroiliitis)
2. arthropathy associated with inflammatory bowel disease (bilateral and symmetrical)
3. psoriatic arthritis (bilateral and asymmetrical)
4. Reiter's syndrome (bilateral and asymmetrical).

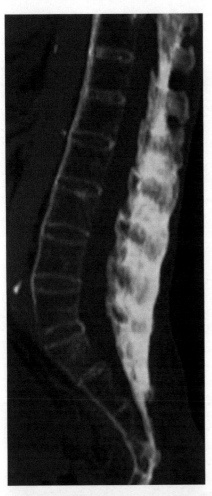

Figure v1.2b: CT showing ossification of anterior longitudinal and interspinous ligaments.

Figure v1.2c: CT showing ankylosis of bilateral sacroiliac joints.

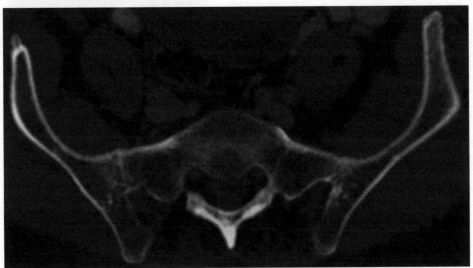

CASE 1.3: 25-YEAR-OLD WITH WEIGHT LOSS

Figure v1.3a

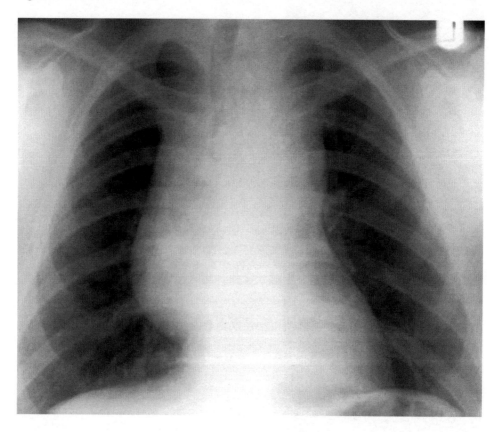

ANTERIOR MEDIASTINAL MASS: LYMPHOMA

FINDINGS

1. Lobulated soft tissue mass causing mediastinal widening.
2. Mass is located more towards the right side of the mediastinum.
3. Anterior junctional line is obliterated.
4. Posterior mediastinal lines are preserved.
5. Right hilum is visible behind the mass.

INTERPRETATION

Findings consistent with an anterior mediastinal mass.

MAIN DIAGNOSIS

Given the history of weight loss, lymphoma is the most likely cause in a patient of this age.

DIFFERENTIAL DIAGNOSIS

1. Germ-cell tumour.
2. Thymic masses.
3. Retrosternal goitre.

There are no exact radiographic features that could distinguish germ-cell tumours or thymic masses from lymphoma. The presence of calcifications/teeth or fat-fluid level helps to distinguish mature teratomas from the other masses. A large retrosternal goitre is probably unlikely in view of the young age of the patient. Retrosternal thyroid masses can also be followed above the level of the clavicles.

FURTHER INVESTIGATIONS AND MANAGEMENT

1. CT scan of thorax, abdomen and pelvis.
2. Referral to oncology/haematology team, depending upon the imaging findings.

FURTHER INFORMATION

The 'hilum overlay' sign is present when the hilum is visible behind a mass. This suggests that the mass does not arise from the hilum, but most probably from the anterior mediastinum. Retrosternal thyroid masses can extend into the middle or posterior mediastinum, obliterating the right paratracheal stripe and causing tracheal deviation. Above the level of the clavicles, the anterior mediastinal masses have an ill-defined lateral margin, whereas the posterior masses have an interface with the lung, giving a sharp lateral margin.

CASE 1.4: 45-YEAR-OLD MAN WITH HIP PAIN

Figure v1.4a

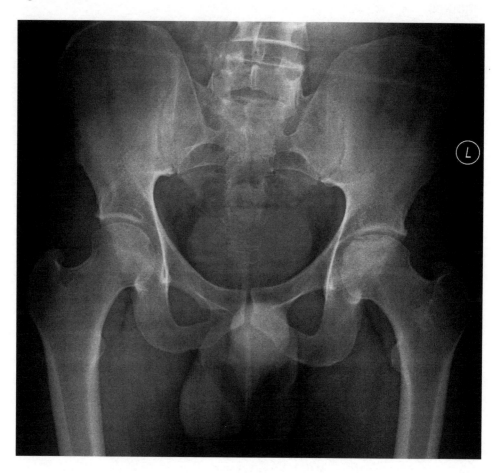

AVASCULAR NECROSIS

FINDINGS

1. Increased sclerosis of the left head of femur.
2. Subchondral patchy lucency at the superior aspect of the left head of femur.
3. Normal joint space and no osteophytes.

DIAGNOSIS

Avascular necrosis of the left femoral head. Causes include the following:
1. steroid intake
2. trauma
3. haemoglobinopathies (e.g. sickle-cell disease)
4. alcoholism
5. pancreatitis
6. Gaucher's disease
7. radiation.

FURTHER INVESTIGATIONS AND MANAGEMENT

1. MRI is indicated to identify any evidence of early avascular necrosis of the right femoral head so that treatment can be instituted prior to the onset of femoral head collapse.
2. Orthopaedic referral for consideration of treatment options to prevent joint damage.

FURTHER INFORMATION

There are a number of causes of avascular necrosis. Sometimes no apparent cause can be identified. In a significant number of patients, avascular necrosis of the hip is bilateral, and therefore both femurs should be imaged. This ensures early detection so that treatment can be instituted prior to any damage occurring to the articular surface. On MRI there is diffuse bone marrow oedema in the early stages, which progresses to a serpiginous T1 low-signal line surrounding an area of fatty marrow. This is the most characteristic sign of avascular necrosis. On T2-weighted images, a heterogeneous high signal can be visualised. In advanced stages, there is a focal low signal on both T1 and T2, consistent with bone collapse and sclerosis.

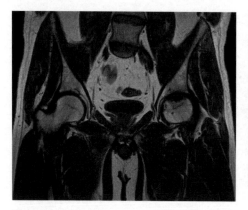 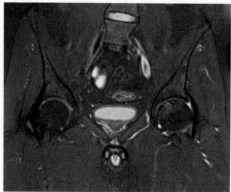

Figures v1.4b and v1.4c: Avascular necrosis of the left head of femur, with low T1 and heterogenous high STIR signal within the superior aspect of the left head of femur. Normal right head of femur.

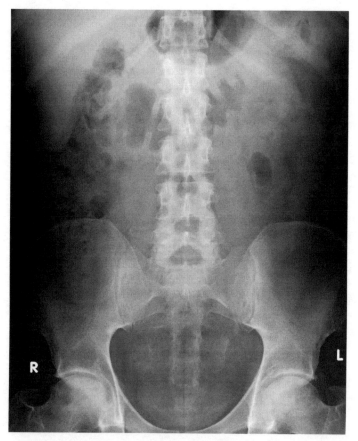

Figure v1.4d: Patient with bilateral avascular necrosis. Note the thickened transverse colonic mucosa. The aetiology is most probably steroid therapy for ulcerative colitis.

CASE 1.5: 30-YEAR-OLD MAN PRESENTING WITH ANKLE SWELLING AND RASH ON THE LEFT SHIN

Figure v1.5a

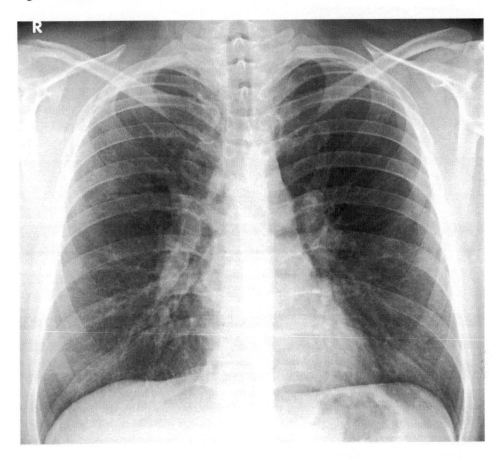

BILATERAL HILAR LYMPHADENOPATHY

FINDINGS

1. Bilateral symmetrical lobulated hilar enlargement.
2. Lungs are clear.

MAIN DIAGNOSIS

Bilateral symmetrical hilar lymph node enlargement, most probably secondary to sarcoidosis. Radiographically, this is stage I sarcoidosis, as there are no pulmonary changes.

DIFFERENTIAL DIAGNOSIS

1. Lymphoma. However, this is less likely because the hilar enlargement is symmetrical and the mediastinal lymph nodes are not enlarged.
2. Tuberculosis. However, this is less likely because the hilar enlargement is bilateral and symmetrical.

FURTHER INVESTIGATIONS AND MANAGEMENT

1. Serum calcium and ACE levels.
2. Referral to the chest team for transbronchial biopsy of enlarged lymph nodes and further medical management.

FURTHER INFORMATION

Bilateral hilar lymph node enlargement is also a common examination case. The differential diagnosis is wide. The points to note are symmetry, any evidence of mediastinal lymph node enlargement and any pulmonary parenchymal changes. Sarcoidosis generally causes bilateral symmetrical lobulated hilar enlargement. With lymphoma, hilar enlargement tends to be asymmetrical and there is often evidence of mediastinal lymph node enlargement. Tuberculosis generally causes unilateral hilar lymph node enlargement. Other conditions such as hypersensitivity pneumonitis and silicosis also produce bilateral hilar enlargement, but there are additional pulmonary parenchymal changes. With pulmonary hypertension the hilar enlargement is smooth.

CASE 1.6: 46-YEAR-OLD MAN WITH CHEST DISCOMFORT

Figure v1.6a

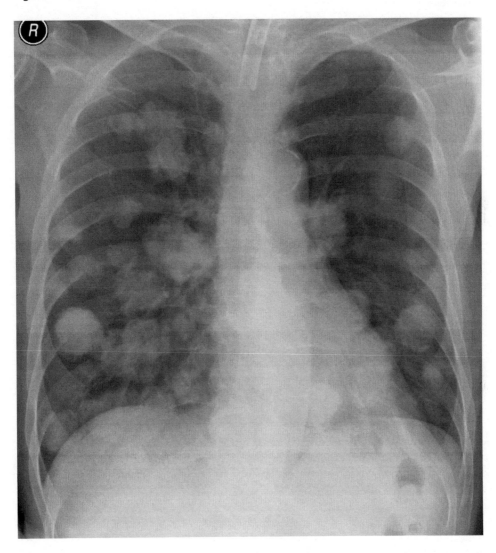

CANNONBALL METASTASES

FINDINGS

1. Multiple bilateral round soft tissue density nodules of various sizes throughout both lungs.
2. No calcification or cavitation.
3. Tracheostomy tube *in situ*.

DIAGNOSIS

Multiple cannonball pulmonary metastases. The primary tumour could be any of the following:
1. seminoma
2. sarcoma
3. colon carcinoma
4. renal-cell carcinoma.

DIFFERENTIAL DIAGNOSES

1. Fungal disease.
2. Wegener's granulomatosis.

In both of these conditions, cavitation can occur in a significant number of patients. Cavitation is less likely in metastases, and most frequently occurs in metastatic squamous-cell carcinoma.

FURTHER INVESTIGATIONS AND MANAGEMENT

1. If primary malignancy is not clinically evident, seminoma and prostate carcinoma must in particular be excluded, as these cancers may respond to a combination of chemotherapy, hormonal therapy and radiotherapy.
2. If there is no obvious primary malignancy, biopsy of one of the lesions is justified to exclude granulomatous and infective causes.

FURTHER INFORMATION

Multiple bilateral pulmonary nodules on chest X-ray are a common examination case. This case mainly tests the candidate's knowledge of the various primary neoplasms that can give rise to multiple large well-defined haematogenous metastases to the lungs (the so-called cannonball metastases). A similar appearance can occur with benign conditions, although these are more likely to cavitate than metastatic disease.

CASE 1.7: ONE-MONTH-OLD INFANT WITH PROGRESSIVE ABDOMINAL DISTENSION

Figure v1.7a

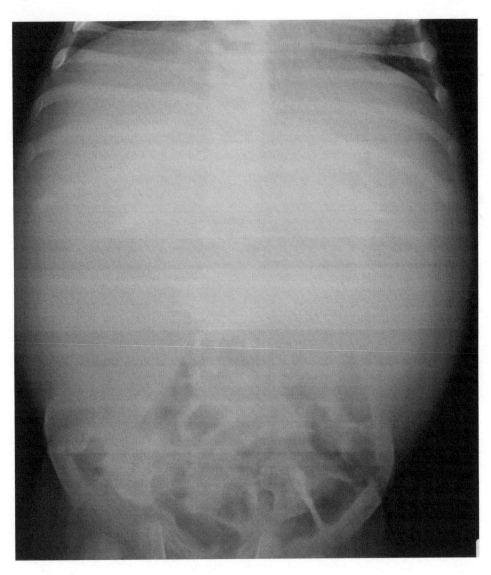

HEPATOSPLENOMEGALY

FINDINGS

1. Soft tissue opacification of the right and left upper quadrants.
2. Medial and inferior displacement of bowel loops.

DIFFERENTIAL DIAGNOSIS

1. Hepatosplenomegaly. Possible causes include the following:
   - haemolytic anaemias (e.g. sickle-cell anaemia, thalassaemia)
   - storage disorders (e.g. Gaucher's disease)
   - infection (e.g. congenital cytomegalovirus, toxoplasma, hepatitis A, B or C)
   - haematological malignancies (e.g. leukaemia, lymphoma).
2. Polycystic kidneys.

FURTHER INVESTIGATIONS AND MANAGEMENT

1. Abdominal ultrasound.
2. Referral to paediatricians for further history, bloods, virology and bone marrow aspiration.

FURTHER INFORMATION

Hepatosplenomegaly in a young child or infant could broadly be due to malignant, metabolic or infective processes.

- Malignant causes: leukaemia, lymphoma, neuroblastoma, Wilms' tumour, hepatoblastoma, hepatocellular carcinoma.
- Metabolic causes: Gaucher's disease, Niemann–Pick disease, Hurler's syndrome, Wilson's disease, haemochromatosis, hypervitaminosis A.
- Infective causes: viral (cytomegalovirus, Epstein–Barr virus, HIV), bacterial (tuberculosis, *Brucella, Bartonella*), fungal (*Candida, Histoplasma*), protozoal (malaria).

CASE 1.8: 76-YEAR-OLD MAN WITH HAEMOPTYSIS

Figure v1.8a

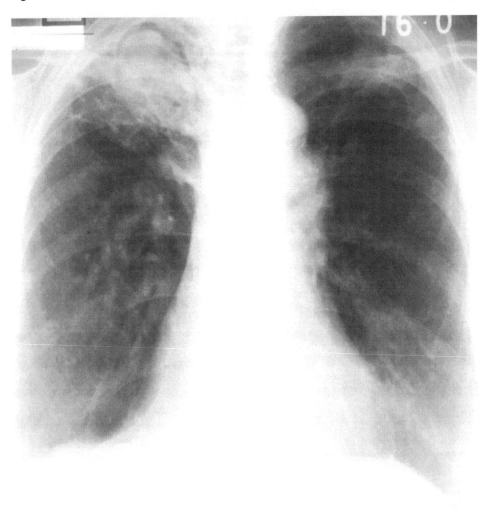

INTRACAVITARY MYCETOMA

FINDINGS

1. Bilateral upper zone volume loss.
2. Bilateral apical scarring which is worse on the right side, where there is also bronchial wall thickening and dilatation consistent with bronchiectasis.
3. Large, thick-walled cavity containing intracavitary soft tissue.
4. Air-crescent sign at the superior aspect of the cavity.

MAIN DIAGNOSIS

Intracavitary mycetoma at the right lung apex in a pre-existing cavity, most probably secondary to previous tuberculosis.

DIFFERENTIAL DIAGNOSIS

Scar carcinoma. However, the presence of an air-crescent sign is typical of an intra-cavitary fungus ball.

FURTHER INVESTIGATIONS AND MANAGEMENT

1. CT thorax.
2. *Aspergillus* precipitins and sputum cultures.
3. Respiratory referral for further treatment.

FURTHER INFORMATION

Aspergilloma is generally found in immunocompetent hosts. Mycetoma is a tangle of fungal hyphae, cellular debris and mucus. It is a mobile mass and lies in a dependent position. Intracavitary mycetoma may cause massive, life-threatening haemoptysis.

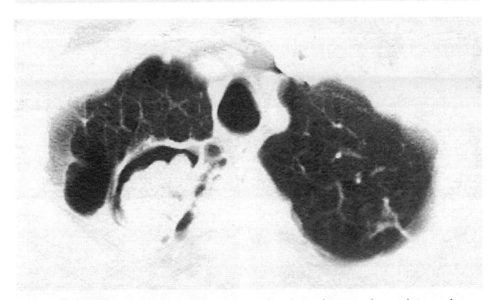

Figure v1.8b: Close-up of the right lung apex showing a large cavity, an intracavitary mycetoma and the air-crescent sign.

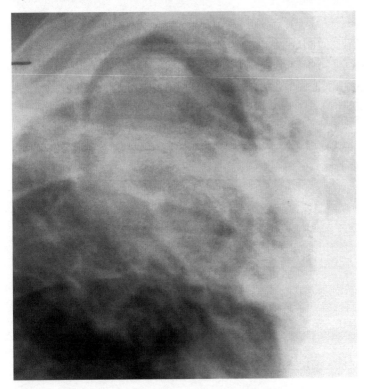

Figure v1.8c: CT showing a fungus ball at the posterior (dependent) aspect of the cavity with air-crescent sign anteriorly.

CASE 1.9: 70-YEAR-OLD MAN WITH BACK PAIN

Figures v1.9a and v1.9b

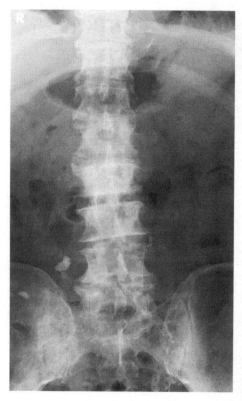

a

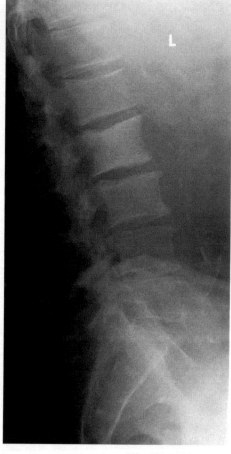

b

IVORY VERTEBRA

FINDINGS

1. Sclerosis of L2 vertebral body – 'ivory vertebra'.
2. The posterior elements are spared.
3. Bridging osteophytosis and disc-space narrowing consistent with lumbar spondylosis.
4. Calcification of the abdominal aorta.

DIFFERENTIAL DIAGNOSIS

1. Sclerotic metastasis, in particular prostate cancer in a male patient.
2. Paget's disease – vertebral body is usually expanded.
3. Lymphoma.

FURTHER INVESTIGATIONS AND MANAGEMENT

1. Detailed clinical history.
2. PSA measurement.
3. Bone scan to look for other sclerotic deposits.
4. CT chest, abdomen and pelvis to look for primary malignancy/lymphoma.

FURTHER INFORMATION

In the so-called 'ivory vertebra' almost the whole of the vertebral body is sclerotic. Osteoblastic metastasis, lymphoma and Paget's disease are the most common causes of an ivory vertebra. Osteoblastic metastases can arise from carcinoma of the prostate, breast, gastrointestinal tract, lung and urinary bladder. In Paget's disease, the vertebral body is usually expanded.

CASE 1.10: 20-YEAR-OLD WITH PAINLESS FINGER SWELLING

Figure v1.10a

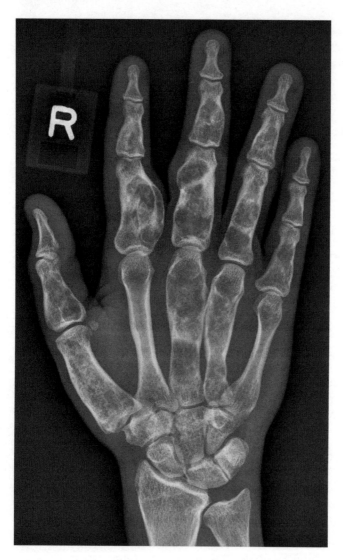

MULTIPLE ENCHONDROMAS

FINDINGS

1. Expansile lytic lesions within multiple metacarpal bones and phalanges, producing bone-modelling deformities.
2. The lesions are located centrally and eccentrically, and randomly distributed in epi-, meta- and diaphyses.
3. Lesions cause endosteal scalloping and cortical thinning.
4. Ill-defined 'dot- and arc-like' matrix mineralisation.
5. Narrrow zone of transition.
6. No periosteal reaction.
7. No soft tissue swelling or calcifications.
8. No pathological fractures.

MAIN DIAGNOSIS

Multiple enchondromas (Ollier's disease).

DIFFERENTIAL DIAGNOSIS

Maffucci's syndrome. However, no soft tissue haemangiomas are visible on this single view of the right hand.

FURTHER INVESTIGATIONS AND MANAGEMENT

1. Search for any soft tissue haemangiomas to exclude Maffucci's syndrome.
2. Orthopaedic referral for further treatment and follow-up.

FURTHER INFORMATION

Ollier's disease is the presence of multiple enchondromas. The risk of malignant transformation in Ollier's disease is approximately 25–30%. Maffucci's syndrome is a combination of multiple enchondromas with soft tissue haemangiomas. Although the incidence of development of malignant degeneration in skeletal lesions is similar in both of these conditions, there is an increased risk of development of non-musculoskeletal malignancies in Maffucci's syndrome. Therefore it is important to distinguish Ollier's disease from Maffucci's syndrome. Development of pain in the skeletal lesions should raise suspicion of malignant degeneration of skeletal lesions in both of these conditions. Malignancies associated with Maffucci's syndrome are gastrointestinal, pancreatic and ovarian cancers, and gliomas.

CASE 1.11: 80-YEAR-OLD MAN WITH RIGHT HIP PAIN

Figure v1.11a

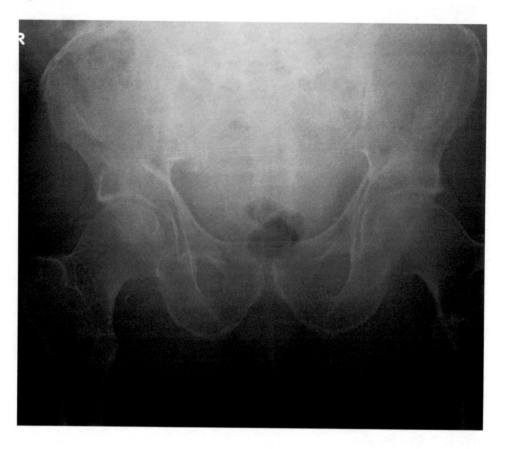

MULTIPLE MYELOMA

FINDINGS

1. Well-defined lytic lesions of bilateral proximal femoral shafts and left neck of femur. Lesions are centred at the medullary cavity.
2. Endosteal scalloping.
3. No pathological fracture.

MAIN DIAGNOSIS

Multiple myeloma.

DIFFERENTIAL DIAGNOSIS

Multiple bone metastases. Endosteal scalloping is more suggestive of myeloma than of metastases. However, as metastases remain a high possibility, the radiological findings must be interpreted in conjunction with serum paraprotein levels.

FURTHER INVESTIGATIONS AND MANAGEMENT

1. Skeletal survey to look for any other lesion.
2. Serum and urine paraproteins, and serum calcium.
3. Haematology review for further management.

FURTHER INFORMATION

Lytic lesions are visible on plain radiographs only after 30% of the bone has been destroyed. Diffuse demineralisation is also a feature of myeloma. Rarely (in 1% of cases) myeloma deposits can be sclerotic, as part of POEMS syndrome (polyneuropathy, organomegaly, endocrinopathy, monoclonal gammopathy and skin changes). Myeloma deposits are low signal on T1- and high signal on T2-weighted MRI, are hot in MDP bone scans in only 10% of cases, and are FDG avid.

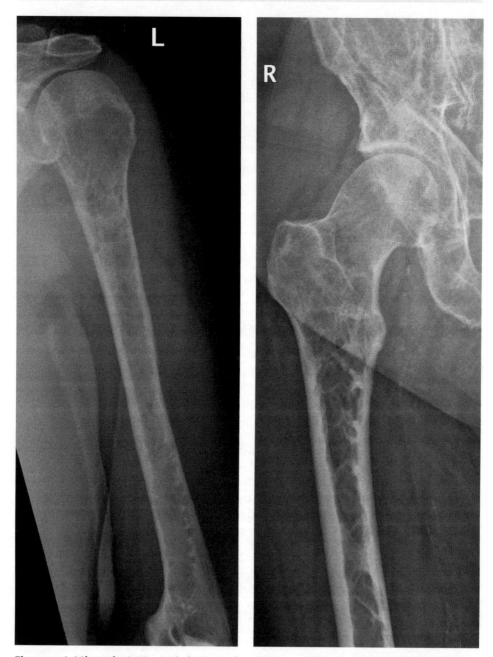

Figures v1.11b and v1.11c: Lytic lesions of multiple myeloma involving the right femur and left humerus in the same patient.

CASE 1.12: 30-YEAR-OLD WOMAN WITH BILATERAL LEG WEAKNESS

Figures v1.12a and v1.12b

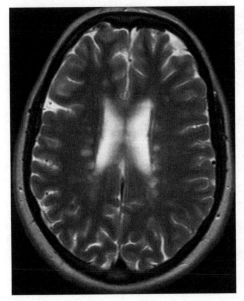
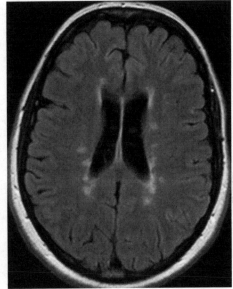

a   b

MULTIPLE SCLEROSIS

FINDINGS

T2 and FLAIR axial MR images through the brain:
1. Multiple bilateral T2 high-signal lesions
2. Lesions are located in the periventricular white matter
3. Most of the individual lesions are ovoid in shape.

MAIN DIAGNOSIS

Multiple sclerosis.

DIFFERENTIAL DIAGNOSIS

1. White matter ischaemia. However, this is unlikely as the patient is young, and the lesions are mainly periventricular and radially orientated.
2. Vasculitides such as SLE. However, in general the periventricular white matter is spared.

FURTHER INVESTIGATIONS AND MANAGEMENT

1. MRI of the whole spine.
2. Neurology referral.

FURTHER INFORMATION

The definite diagnosis of multiple sclerosis is based on two or more episodes of symptoms and two or more signs that reflect involvement of at least two non-contiguous white matter tracts of the CNS. At least one of the signs must be on clinical examination and the other may be on a paraclinical test (MRI or visual, auditory or somatosensory evoked potential). On MRI, the MS plaques appear as radially orientated ovoid periventricular T2 high-signal lesions. Lesions may also be detected on optic nerves, corpus callosum, cerebellar peduncles, brainstem and spinal cord. Large lesions causing mass effect are called tumefactive plaques. Acute MS plaques can enhance on post-Gd images. Tumefactive plaques demonstrate an incomplete ring enhancement. Long-standing MS can cause cerebral and spinal cord atrophy.

CASE 1.13: 57-YEAR-OLD MALE SMOKER WITH COUGH

Figure v1.13a

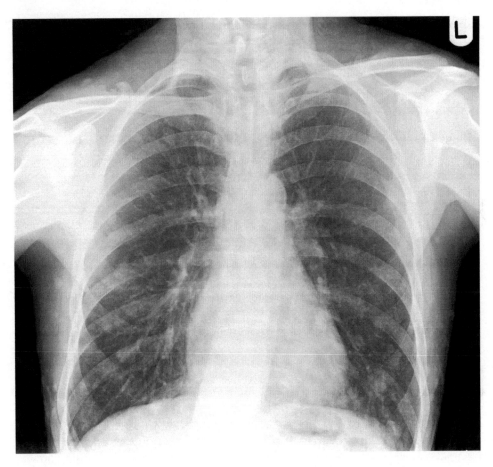

NEUROFIBROMATOSIS

FINDINGS

1. Multiple rounded soft tissue density opacities projected throughout the thorax.
2. Some of these opacities projected outwith the lungs in the soft tissues of axillae and supraclavicular regions.
3. No rib anomaly identified.

INTERPRETATION

Multiple well-defined soft tissue skin lesions.

DIAGNOSIS

Multiple cutaneous neurofibromas.

FURTHER INVESTIGATIONS AND MANAGEMENT

1. Clinical examination to confirm the presence of multiple cutaneous neurofibromas.
2. As the presence of intrapulmonary neoplastic lesions cannot be excluded on the basis of the chest X-ray, CT scan is necessary, given the patient's presenting symptoms.

FURTHER INFORMATION

Neurofibromas are benign peripheral nerve tumours that present as multiple cutaneous nodules. Cutaneous neurofibromas occur commonly in NF-1 but rarely in NF-2. Café-au-lait spots, axillary freckling, iris hamartomas, pseudarthrosis of tibia, sphenoid wing dysplasia, spinal neurofibromas, scoliosis and rib notching are other features of NF-1. NF-1 patients are at increased risk of developing plexiform neurofibromas, optic pathway gliomas, ependymomas, meningiomas, astrocytomas and phaeochromocytomas. Bilateral vestibular schwannomas are characteristic of NF-2, occuring in over 90% of individuals who carry the NF-2 gene. NF-2 patients are also at risk of developing meningiomas, gliomas, and schwannomas of cranial and spinal nerves. Juvenile posterior subcapsular cataract is also characteristic of NF-2.

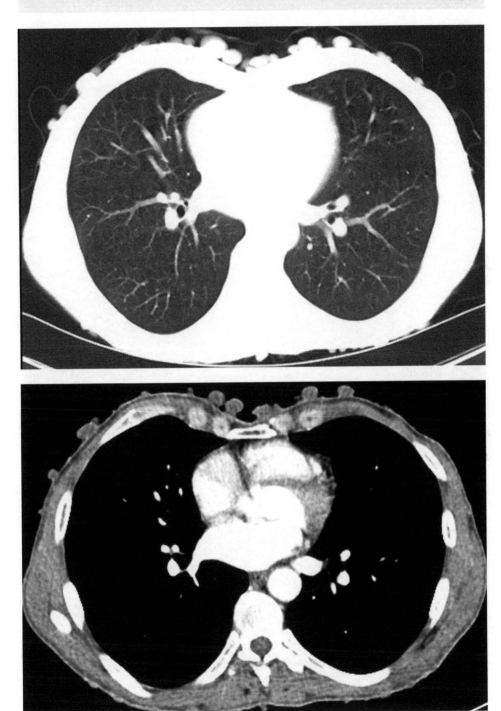

Figures v1.13b and v1.13c: CT scan showing multiple cutaneous soft tissue nodules consistent with neurofibromas.

CASE 1.14: INFANT PRESENTING WITH ANKLE SWELLING

Figures v1.14a and v1.14b

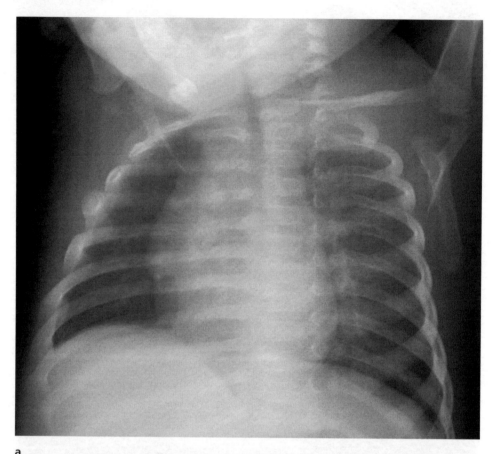

a

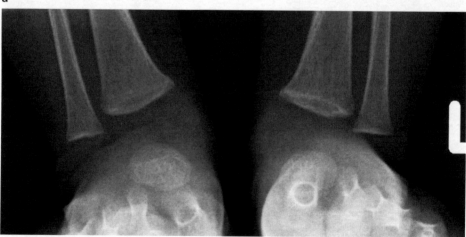

b

NON-ACCIDENTAL INJURY

FINDINGS

1. Chest X-ray:
   a. Acute fractures of the left fifth and sixth ribs posteriorly
   b. Healing fracture of the right fourth rib laterally.
2. X-ray ankles:
   a. Left tibial metaphyseal corner fracture.

MAIN DIAGNOSIS

Non-accidental injury.

DIFFERENTIAL DIAGNOSIS

1. Accidental traumatic fractures. However, this is unlikely as there are fractures of varying ages.
2. Osteogenesis imperfecta. However, this is unlikely as metaphyseal corner fractures are rare with osteogenesis imperfecta. There is also no evidence of osteopaenia or cortical thinning.

FURTHER INVESTIGATIONS AND MANAGEMENT

1. Alert the physicians to take a careful history and examination.
2. Involve social services.
3. Perform a complete skeletal survey.
4. In acute presentation with head injury, CT with or without MRI is required, looking for subdural and subarachnoid haemorrhage, brain oedema, contusions and axonal shearing injury (particularly pericallosal). MRI is needed if presentation is non-acute.

FURTHER INFORMATION

Skeletal hallmarks of non-accidental injury are as follows:
- fractures at different stages of healing
- metaphyseal corner fractures or bucket-handle fractures, usually around the wrists or ankles, relating to periosteal avulsion
- posterior rib fractures
- long bone spiral fractures in children who are not walking
- depressed skull fractures
- scapula or spinous process fractures.

CASE 1.15: 80-YEAR-OLD MAN WITH WEIGHT LOSS

Figure v1.15a

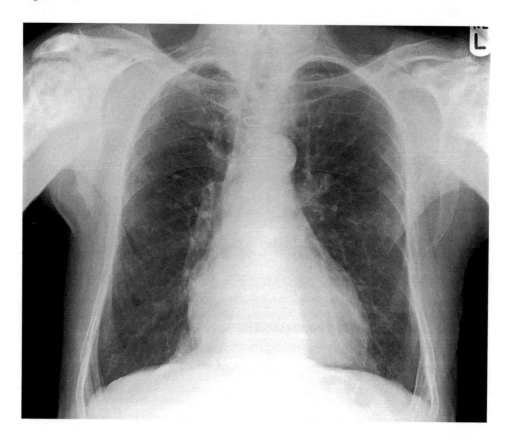

PAGET'S DISEASE

FINDINGS

1. Previous sternotomy with evidence of coronary bypass surgery.
2. Borderline cardiomegaly but normal pulmonary vascularity.
3. No focal lung lesion.
4. Cortical thickening, coarse trabecular pattern and sclerosis within both proximal humeri.
5. Sclerosis of right scapula.

MAIN DIAGNOSIS

Paget's disease.

DIFFERENTIAL DIAGNOSIS

Osteoblastic metastases. However, subarticular involvement and coarse trabecular pattern are features that support Paget's disease.

FURTHER INVESTIGATIONS AND MANAGEMENT

1. Image the whole of both forearms.
2. A bone scan may be useful for obtaining an overview of the skeleton, and for assessing change or malignant degeneration.
3. Alkaline phosphatase, which is high in Paget's disease.
4. Serum PSA and acid phosphatase, which are high in prostate secondaries.

FURTHER INFORMATION

Paget's disease is characterised by bone resorption followed by immature bone deposition. There are lytic, mixed lytic–sclerotic and sclerotic phases of the disease. In the lytic phase there are flame-shaped lytic areas, particularly in the subarticular location. This is followed by coarsening of primary trabeculae and cortical thickening, leading to loss of the normal corticomedullary junction. Osteoporosis circumscripta, cotton wool sclerosis, expansion of the diploic space and foraminal narrowing are features of Paget's disease in the skull. 'Picture-frame vertebra' and bowing of the tibia are other features of Paget's disease.

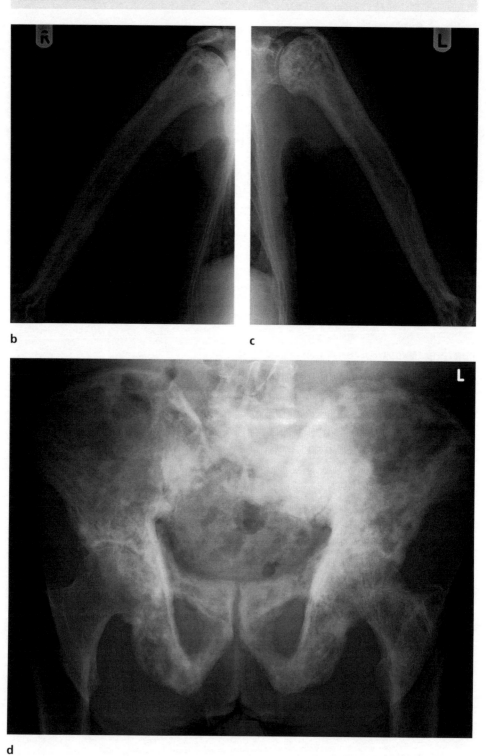

b

c

d

Figures v1.15b, 1.15c and 1.15d: Paget's disease of both arms and pelvis.

CASE 1.16: 60-YEAR-OLD MAN WITH SHORTNESS OF BREATH AND RESTRICTIVE RESPIRATORY DEFECT

Figure v1.16a

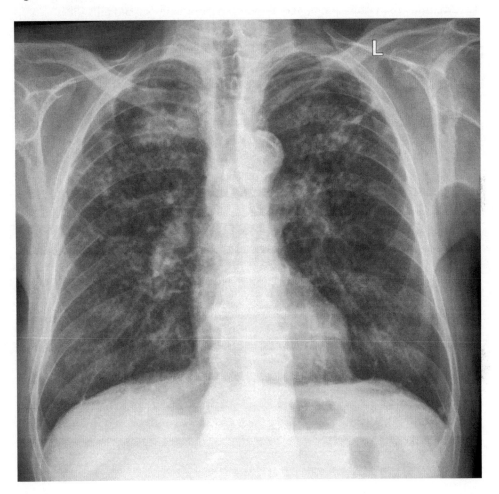

PROGRESSIVE MASSIVE FIBROSIS

FINDINGS

1. Multiple small dense pulmonary nodules within the upper and mid zones bilaterally.
2. Coalescing nodules in both upper zones, forming ill defined but relatively symmetrical masses.
3. Bilateral superior hilar traction consistent with upper lobe volume loss.

DIAGNOSIS

Progressive massive fibrosis (PMF) against a background of pneumoconiosis, most probably silicosis.

FURTHER INVESTIGATIONS AND MANAGEMENT

1. Review previous radiographs.
2. Determine occupational history.
3. Referral to the respiratory team.

FURTHER INFORMATION

PMF complicates pneumoconiosis and is more commonly seen in patients with a history of silica dust exposure. The large coalescent masses in the upper zones should not be confused with bronchogenic carcinoma. These masses show very slow progression on serial radiographs. The apical masses are typically symmetrical. As the disease progresses, these masses migrate towards the hila and cause a reduction in background pulmonary nodularity due to coalescence of nodules into the fibrotic masses. There is also peripheral compensatory emphysema. The masses of PMF may sometimes cavitate secondary to central necrosis or coexisting tuberculosis – this should prompt further investigations. The condition is progressive, and death is usually due to cor pulmonale and respiratory failure.

CASE 1.17: 82-YEAR-OLD WOMAN WITH ACUTE-ONSET LEFT LOWER QUADRANT PAIN AND SWELLING

Figures v1.17a and v1.17b

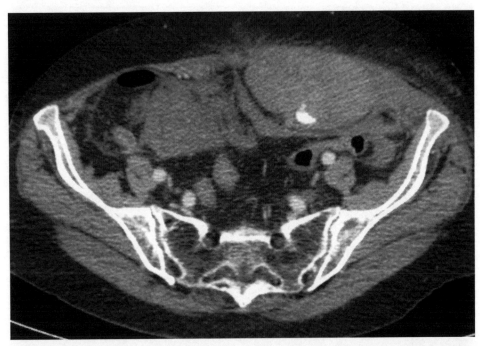

a

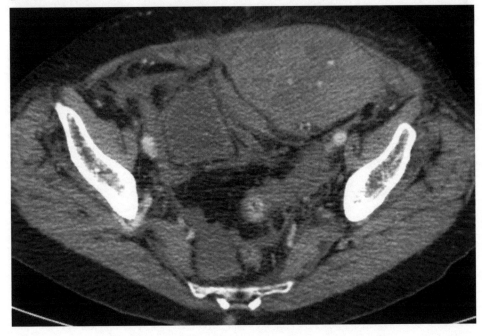

b

RECTUS SHEATH HAEMATOMA

FINDINGS

Post-contrast CT abdomen:
1. Large high-attenuation oval mass that is inseparable from the left rectus abdominis muscle
2. Inferior epigastric vessels displaced posteriorly
3. High-density contrast blush at the inferior aspect of the mass
4. Mass does not cross midline, and right rectus abdominis muscle appears normal
5. Bowel loops displaced posteriorly by the mass
6. Stranding in the deep subcutaneous fat in the left anterior abdominal wall
7. Free fluid within the pelvis.

MAIN DIAGNOSIS

Large left rectus sheath haematoma with active contrast extravasation from a left inferior epigastric vessel.

DIFFERENTIAL DIAGNOSIS

1. Desmoid tumour. However, this is unlikely as this tumour mainly occurs in women of childbearing age.
2. Malignancy – sarcoma and metastasis. However, acute-onset pain and swelling are features that argue against these diagnoses.

FURTHER INVESTIGATIONS AND MANAGEMENT

1. Immediate surgical referral.
2. Interventional radiology consultation for potential embolisation.
3. Explore history of anticoagulant therapy or trauma.

FURTHER INFORMATION

Rectus sheath haematomas are most often related to anticoagulant treatment. They are often accompanied by a rapid decline in haematocrit, and by abdominal swelling and skin discoloration. Rectus sheath haematomas are limited to one side by the linea alba in the midline. Large haematomas can extend into the pelvis below the level of the arcuate line and compress the pelvic viscera.

CASE 1.18: ABDOMINAL DISTENSION

Figure v1.18a

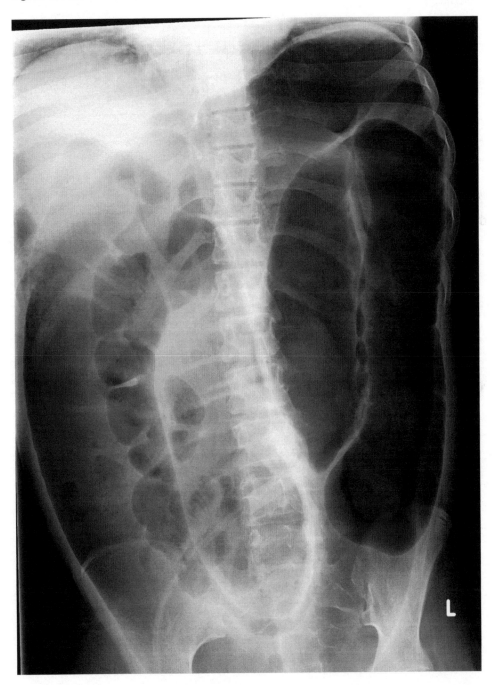

SIGMOID VOLVULUS

FINDINGS

1. Marked distension of the large bowel loops.
2. A 'coffee bean'-shaped loop of distended ahaustral large bowel arising from the pelvis.
3. Distended descending colon.
4. Small bowel not distended.
5. No free gas.

MAIN DIAGNOSIS

Sigmoid volvulus.

DIFFERENTIAL DIAGNOSIS

Caecal volvulus. However, the distension of the descending colon argues against this diagnosis.

FURTHER INVESTIGATIONS AND MANAGEMENT

1. Surgical referral for further management.
2. If there is any doubt about the plain radiographic appearances, a water-soluble contrast enema can be used to confirm the diagnosis.

FURTHER INFORMATION

Sigmoid volvulus often occurs in elderly mentally debilitated patients, and the condition may be chronic or intermittent. On plain radiograph, sigmoid volvulus appears as a disproportionately distended ahaustral loop of large bowel. The shape is an inverted 'U', which is classically described as 'coffee bean' shaped. Liver overlap sign and descending colon overlap sign may also be present. On water-soluble enema study, sigmoid volvulus appears as a smooth tapered narrowing of the sigmoid colon giving rise to a 'bird of prey' appearance.

Caecal volvulus often occurs in young patients. When the caecum twists, it lies in the axial plane and the distended loop is visualised in the right lower quadrant or central abdomen. When the caecum twists and inverts, the distended loop is visualised in the left upper quadrant. Haustral markings in the caecum can still be appreciated; the left colon collapses and the small bowel may be distended.

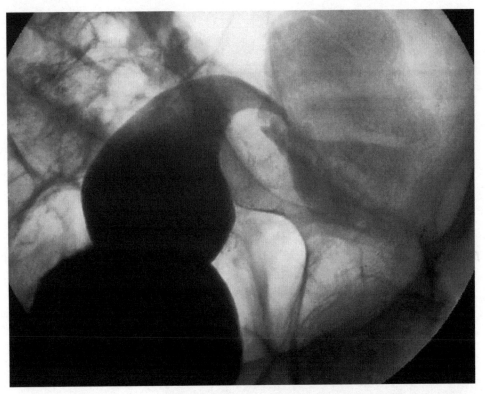

Figure 1.18b: 'Bird of prey' appearance of sigmoid volvulus on water-soluble contrast enema.

CASE 1.19: 49-YEAR-OLD WOMAN WITH COELIAC DISEASE

Figures v1.19a and v1.19b

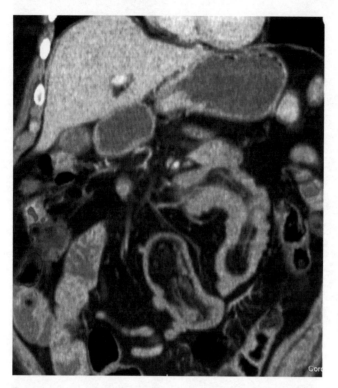

a

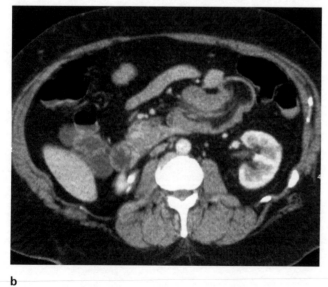

b

ENTERO-ENTERIC INTUSSUSCEPTION

FINDINGS

1. Long segment of small bowel wall thickening and distension.
2. Intraluminal fat and linear structures consistent with mesenteric fat and mesenteric vessels.
3. No lymph node enlargement in the visualised images.

DIAGNOSIS

Entero-enteric intussusception. No evidence of small bowel obstruction.

FURTHER INVESTIGATIONS AND MANAGEMENT

1. Against a background of coeliac disease, small bowel lymphoma as the cause of intussusception must be considered, and barium follow-through or MRI of the small bowel should be considered.
2. If features of small bowel obstruction develop, surgical resection may be necessary.

FURTHER INFORMATION

Short-segment entero-enteric intussusceptions in an adult are generally not significant, but long-segment intussusceptions, especially if they are causing small bowel obstruction, must be further evaluated to exclude a tumour acting as a lead point. Similarly, colonic intussusceptions must also be evaluated to exclude a tumour.

Radiological findings of coeliac disease include small bowel wall thickening, jejunisation of ileum or jejunoileal fold pattern reversal, benign lymph node enlargement and free fluid. Entero-enteric intussusception in coeliac disease is generally transient and non-obstructive. However, there is an increased risk of small bowel lymphoma in coeliac disease, and any clinical suspicion should prompt further imaging.

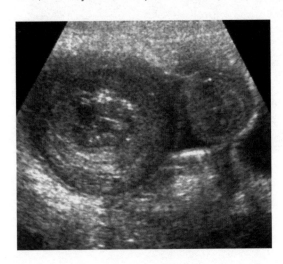

Figure v1.19c: Intussusception: target sign in ultrasound.

CASE 1.20: 45-YEAR-OLD WOMAN WITH SEVERE HEADACHE

Figures v1.20a, v1.20b, v1.20c and v1.20d

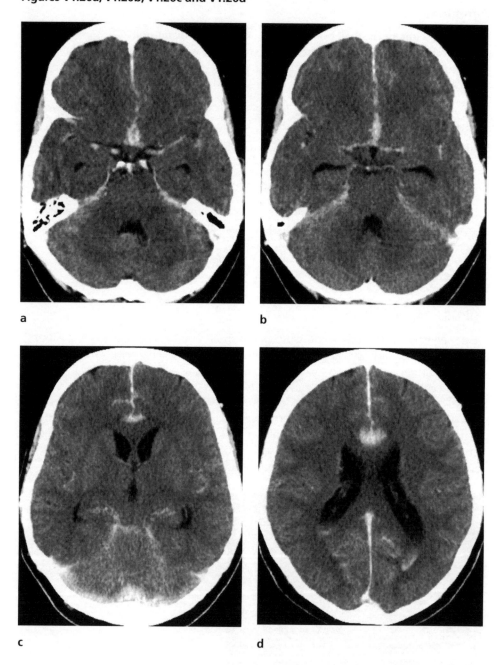

a

b

c

d

SUBARACHNOID HAEMORRHAGE

FINDINGS

Non-contrast CT scan of brain:
1. High attenuation within the interhemispheric fissure, cerebral sulci, Sylvian fissures and quadrigeminal plate cistern, and above the tentorium
2. Early dilatation of the temporal horns of the lateral ventricles and the third ventricle
3. No infarction.

DIAGNOSIS

Subarachnoid haemorrhage complicated by early hydrocephalus. The cause is most probably rupture of a berry aneurysm.

FURTHER INVESTIGATIONS AND MANAGEMENT

1. CT angiography.
2. Referral to the neurology and neuroradiology team with a view to digital subtraction angiography and coiling of the aneurysm.

FURTHER INFORMATION

The possible causes of subarachnoid haemorrhage are trauma, rupture of a berry aneurysm, arteriovenous malformation, blood dyscrasia or bleeding into tumours. Leakage of blood into the subarachnoid space can also occur as a result of intraparenchymal haemorrhage. Repeat angiography may be necessary in patients with angiographically negative subarachnoid haemorrhage, as sometimes the initial angiography may be falsely negative secondary to spasm. Non-aneurysmal perimesencephalic haemorrhage has a benign clinical course. Rebleeding, hydrocephalus and vasospasm leading to infarction are the acute complications of subarachnoid haemorrhage.

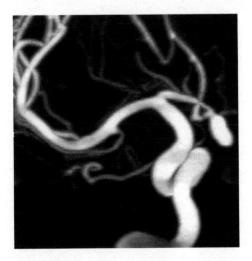

Figure v1.20e: MIP image showing a large anterior communicating artery aneurysm.

CASE 1.21: SHORTNESS OF BREATH

Figure v1.21a

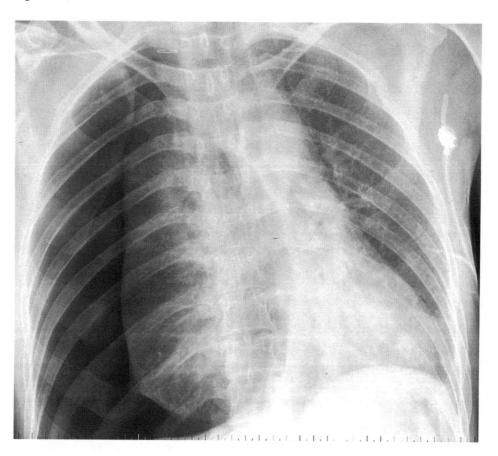

TENSION PNEUMOTHORAX

FINDINGS

1. Large right pneumothorax.
2. Mediastinal shift to the left.
3. Depression of the right hemidiaphragm.

DIAGNOSIS

Tension pneumothorax.

FURTHER INVESTIGATIONS AND MANAGEMENT

Emergency intrathoracic drain insertion.

FURTHER INFORMATION

Tension pneumothorax is a medical emergency. As tension builds up, the venous return to the heart is diminished, and hence the cardiac output. If left untreated, the condition is lethal. Signs of tension pneumothorax are displacement of mediastinum to the opposite side, and depression of the ipsilateral hemidiaphragm. The former sign is more reliable than the latter. However, it is worth noting that tension pneumothorax is a clinical diagnosis, and, if suspected, it must be treated urgently.

A supine pneumothorax can be very subtle, and a high index of suspicion is necessary for the diagnosis. A hyperlucent upper abdominal quadrant, sharply defined costophrenic or cardiophrenic angles, and sharply defined dome of diaphragm or cardiac border are signs of pneumothorax on a supine radiograph.

CASE 1.22: DIARRHOEA AND BLEEDING PER RECTUM

Figure v1.22a

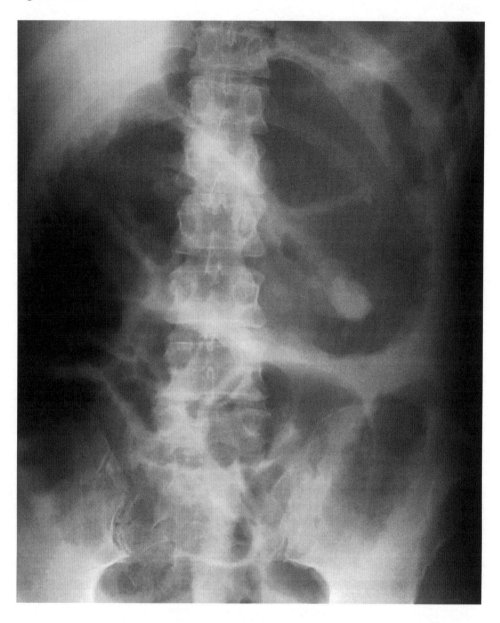

TOXIC MEGACOLON

FINDINGS

1. Diffusely abnormal colonic mucosa with loss of haustral markings.
2. Extensive thickening and irregularity of the colonic mucosa.
3. A distended, empty colon.
4. Free gas visualised within the left upper quadrant.
5. Normal sacroiliac joints.

MAIN DIAGNOSIS

Toxic megacolon with colonic perforation, most probably secondary to ulcerative colitis.

DIFFERENTIAL DIAGNOSIS

1. Crohn's colitis. However, this is less likely as the colonic involvement is so diffuse.
2. Ischaemic colitis. However, this is less likely as the colonic involvement is so diffuse.
3. Infective colitis, including pseudomembranous colitis. However, there would be a history of previous antibiotic use.

FURTHER INVESTIGATIONS AND MANAGEMENT

Immediate surgical referral.

FURTHER INFORMATION

Toxic dilatation most commonly occurs with ulcerative colitis, and the patient is usually systemically unwell. Ulceration is transmural, causing neuromuscular damage that leads to persistent dilatation. Colonic perforation and peritonitis can occur. Barium enema is contraindicated if toxic dilatation is suspected.

CASE 1.23: SHORTNESS OF BREATH

Figure v1.23a

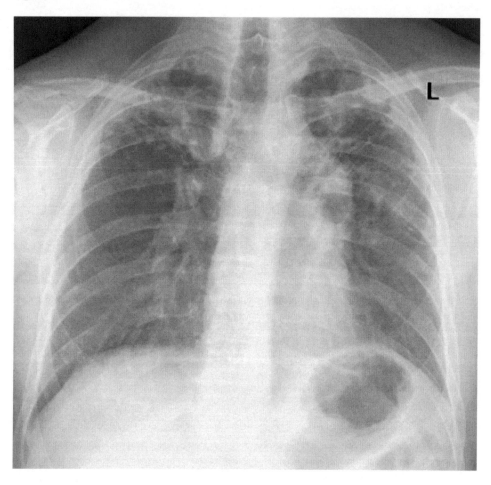

UPPER ZONE FIBROSIS: CHRONIC HYPERSENSITIVITY PNEUMONITIS

FINDINGS

1. Bilateral upper zone volume loss with elevation of both hila.
2. Bilateral upper zone coarse reticulo-nodular opacification.

DIFFERENTIAL DIAGNOSIS

This is broad and includes the following five main conditions.
1. Previous tuberculosis. However, the changes are symmetrical and there are no calcified granulomata.
2. Sarcoidosis. However, there is no bilateral symmetrical hilar lymph node enlargement or calcification.
3. Silicosis. However, there are no calcified lymph nodes, and nodular opacities are not the predominant finding.
4. Chronic hypersensitivity pneumonitis.
5. Ankylosing spondylitis. However, there is no obvious spinal fusion.

FURTHER INVESTIGATIONS AND MANAGEMENT

1. History of exposure to allergens or drugs, and occupation.
2. Review of previous chest X-rays.
3. HRCT.
4. Respiratory team review.

FURTHER INFORMATION

Upper zone pulmonary fibrosis is a common viva case. The differential diagnosis is wide, as outlined above, and pertinent negative findings must be mentioned. This was a case of chronic hypersensitivity pneumonitis. On HRCT there is end-stage fibrosis, characterised by interstitial thickening, traction bronchiectasis or bronchiolectasis, architectural distortion and honeycombing. There may be superimposed subacute ground-glass changes, ill-defined nodularity and air trapping. The lung bases are relatively spared.

The differential diagnosis of upper zone pulmonary fibrosis can be remembered by using the acronym TEARSS:
1. **T**uberculosis. Calcified granulomata and calcified lymph nodes are generally present. Changes are generally asymmetrical.
2. Chronic hypersensitivity pneumonitis (also called extrinsic allergic alveolitis, **E**AA). There may be a history of chronic exposure to an allergen.
3. **A**nkylosing spondylitis. Syndesmophytes and ossified interspinous ligaments may be visualised on CXR.
4. **R**adiation fibrosis. This is related to previous radiation port, but generally upper zone predominant. It is usually unilateral. Look for signs of previous mastectomy.
5. **S**arcoidosis. Bilateral symmetrical hilar lymphadenopathy may be present.
6. **S**ilicosis (pneumoconiosis). There will be a relevant occupational history. Look for conglomerate masses of progressive massive fibrosis.
7. Drug related (gold or nitrofurantoin).

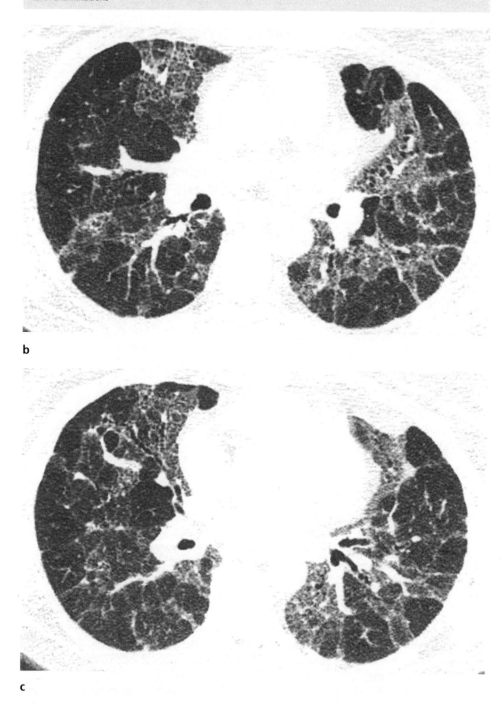

b

c

Figures v1.23b and v1.23c: HRCT showing features of chronic hypersensitivity pneumonitis characterised by architectural distortion, irregular reticular opacification, and traction bronchiectasis and bronchiolectasis. There is also a superimposed subacute ground-glass change.

Viva 2

CASE 2.1: DIARRHOEA AND WEIGHT LOSS

Figure v2.1a

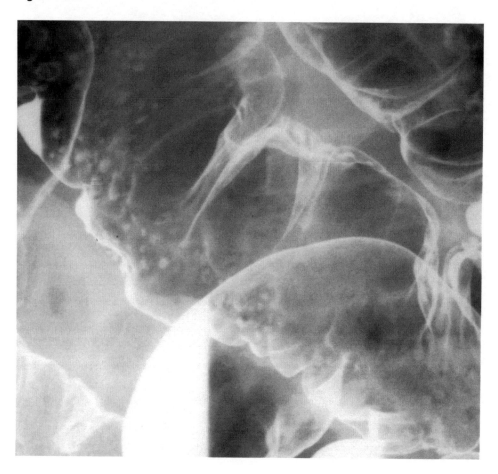

APHTHOID ULCERS IN CROHN'S COLITIS

FINDINGS

Double-contrast barium enema study:
1. Multiple small round ulcers clustered along the transverse colon
2. Lucent halo of oedematous mucosa surrounding the ulcers.

INTERPRETATION

Appearance consistent with multiple colonic aphthoid ulcers.

MAIN DIAGNOSIS

Crohn's disease.

DIFFERENTIAL DIAGNOSIS

1. Tuberculosis.
2. Amoebiasis.
3. Behçet's disease.

Aphthoid ulcers are non-specific and can also occur in the above-mentioned conditions. However, all of these conditions are rare in the UK population.

FURTHER INVESTIGATIONS AND MANAGEMENT

1. Imaging of small bowel to look for small bowel involvement.
2. Search for skip lesions and perianal disease.
3. Gastroenterology referral for endoscopy/biopsy and further medical management.

FURTHER INFORMATION

Aphthoid ulcers are the earliest radiological sign of Crohn's disease. Infections such as tuberculosis and amoebiasis, and inflammatory conditions such as Behçet's disease can also produce aphthoid ulceration, but these conditions are rare in the Western European population. However, aphthoid ulcers do not occur in ulcerative colitis. Behçet's disease is associated with HLA-B51, and clinical manifestations include oral ulcers, skin lesions, genital ulcers, uveitis, recurrent venous thrombosis and a range of neurological involvement. Colonic aphthoid ulcers have been reported in Japanese patients with Behçet's disease. Gastrointestinal tuberculosis is most commonly manifested in the small bowel and caecum. Tuberculosis can produce ulcers, fistulae and anal fistulae – features that simulate Crohn's disease. The chronic form of amoebic colitis clinically resembles inflammatory bowel disease. As steroids can potentiate fulminant forms of amoebic colitis, in areas of high incidence it is important to exclude amoebiasis when inflammatory bowel disease is suspected.

CASE 2.2: 48-YEAR-OLD WOMAN PRESENTING WITH PAIN IN RIGHT RIBS AND BOTH HIPS

Figure v2.2a

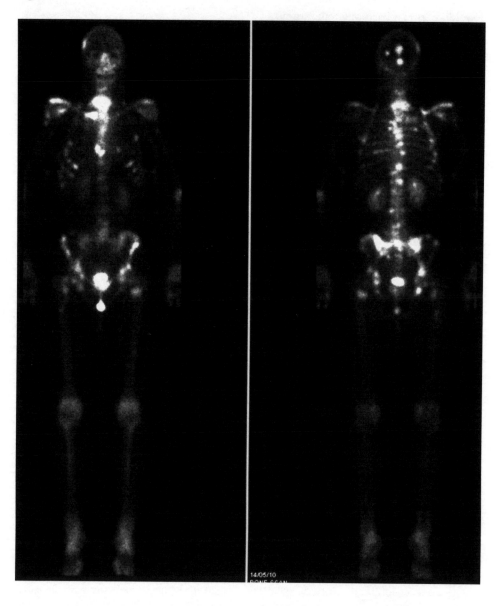

BONE METASTASES

FINDINGS

Radionuclide bone scan of the whole body:
1. Multiple areas of increased radioisotope uptake within the skull vault, throughout the spine, both clavicles, multiple bilateral ribs, bilateral pelvic bones and proximal femora
2. Bilateral breast implants.

INTERPRETATION

Multiple hot spots throughout the bony skeleton in a patient who has bilateral breast implants.

DIAGNOSIS

Multiple bone metastases, most probably secondary to breast carcinoma.

FURTHER INVESTIGATIONS AND MANAGEMENT

1. If there was no previous knowledge of the bone metastases, the patient will also require CT thorax and abdomen to look for visceral and nodal metastases.
2. Oncology referral for palliative therapy.

FURTHER INFORMATION

Bone scans may occasionally be shown in the actual examination. This is a 'classical' case of bone metastases – randomly distributed hot spots throughout the skeleton. Clues such as breast implants, unilateral nephrectomy and an indwelling urinary catheter may point to the primary malignancy. Other conditions, such as multiple traumatic rib fractures or stress fracture of the sacrum, can have classical bone scan appearances, and it is well worth familiarising yourself with them.

CASE 2.3: TWISTED KNEE DURING A FOOTBALL MATCH

Figures v2.3a, 2.3b, 2.3c, 2.3d, 2.3e and 2.3f

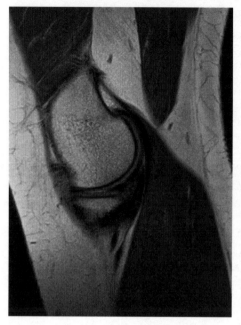

a

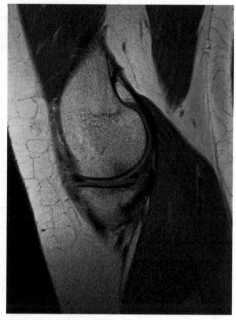

b

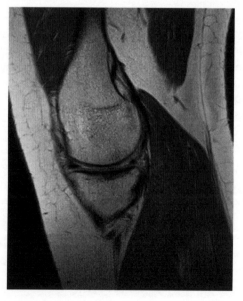

c

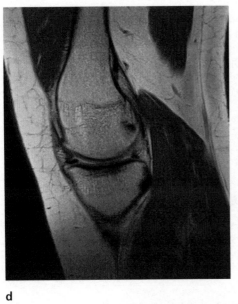

d

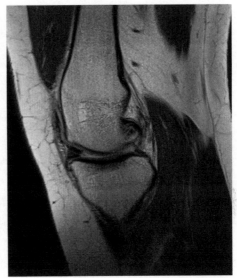

e

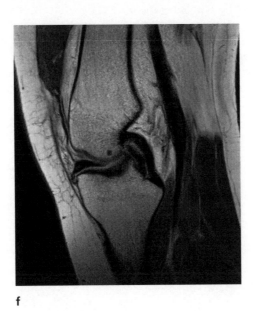

f

BUCKET-HANDLE TEAR

FINDINGS

Sagittal T1-weighted images:
1. Truncation of inner edge of the medial meniscus with loss of normal 'bow-tie' appearance (absent 'bow-tie' sign)
2. Linear low-signal structure parallel and anterior to the posterior cruciate ligament (double PCL sign)
3. Normal posterior cruciate ligament.

DIAGNOSIS

Bucket-handle tear of the medial meniscus.

FURTHER INVESTIGATIONS AND MANAGEMENT

Orthopaedic referral for arthroscopic surgery.

FURTHER INFORMATION

A normal medial or lateral meniscus has a width of approximately 9–12 mm. On sagittal images with a slice thickness of 4–5 mm, a normal meniscus has two contiguous 'bow-ties', and the posterior horn of either meniscus is never smaller than the anterior horn. An absent 'bow-tie' sign is the most reliable indicator of bucket-handle tear. Other conditions in which there is absence of two normal 'bow-ties' are radial tear, degenerative disease of the knee, small/paediatric knee and previous knee surgery. When more than three bow-ties are present, a discoid meniscus must be suspected. The lateral meniscus is more commonly affected by a discoid meniscus, and there is increased risk of meniscal tear.

CASE 2.4: 50-YEAR-OLD WOMAN WITH ABDOMINAL DISCOMFORT

Figures v2.4a, v2.4b, v2.4c and v2.4d

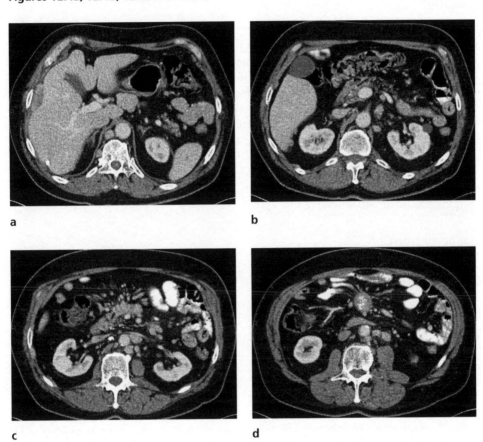

a

b

c

d

CARCINOID TUMOUR

FINDINGS

CT abdomen:
1. Partly calcified soft tissue mesenteric mass
2. Linear stranding radiating from the mass in a 'spoke-wheel' fashion, consistent with desmoplastic reaction
3. Multiple small mesenteric lymph nodes around the mass
4. Multiple enlarged para-aortic and retrocrural lymph nodes
5. Nodularity of the postero-inferior edge of the liver and soft tissue nodules scalloping the lateral and posterior aspect of the right lobe of liver, consistent with peritoneal deposits
6. Coarse calcification at the posterior edge of the right lobe of liver
7. A simple cyst at the midpole of the left kidney
8. Normal liver and adrenals.

MAIN DIAGNOSIS

Carcinoid tumour with multiple peritoneal deposits and enlarged para-aortic, retro-crural and mesenteric lymph nodes.

DIFFERENTIAL DIAGNOSIS

1. Sclerosing mesenteritis.
2. Treated lymphoma.
3. Previous tuberculosis.

All of the above conditions can give rise to a calcified mesenteric mass. However, treated lymphoma and tuberculosis would be known from the previous history. The presence of multiple peritoneal deposits argues against sclerosing mesenteritis and previous tuberculosis.

FURTHER INVESTIGATIONS AND MANAGEMENT

1. Imaging of the thorax and pelvis to assess for further peritoneal, nodal and metastatic disease.
2. Surgical referral.

FURTHER INFORMATION

Carcinoid is the most common primary small bowel tumour. The primary tumour is often submucosal, small and not readily identified on CT. The typical CT appearance is that of a partly calcified mesenteric nodal mass with desmoplastic reaction. The adjacent small bowel loops can be thickened and sometimes kinked. Carcinoid syndrome is the result of metastases to the liver, when the liver becomes unable to metabolise the vasoactive amines, serotonin and tryptophan. Carcinoid liver metastases are typically hypervascular, and bone metastases are osteoblastic. Sclerosing mesenteritis is an idiopathic inflammatory disorder, often associated with other idiopathic inflammatory disorders such as retroperitoneal fibrosis, sclerosing cholangitis, Riedel's thyroiditis and orbital pseudotumour. On CT, there is often preservation of a halo of fat around the affected mesenteric vessels (fat-ring sign).

CASE 2.5: 29-YEAR-OLD WOMAN WITH HEADACHE

Figure v2.5a

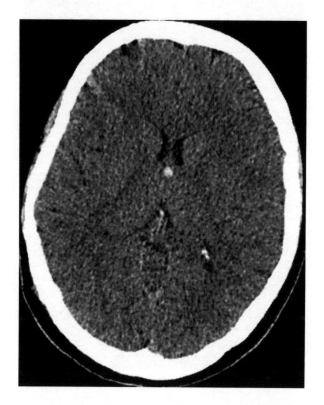

COLLOID CYST OF THE THIRD VENTRICLE

FINDINGS

1. Small high-attenuation rounded mass at the level of foramen of Monro.
2. No ventricular dilatation.

MAIN DIAGNOSIS

Colloid cyst of the third ventricle.

DIFFERENTIAL DIAGNOSIS

Subependymal giant-cell astrocytoma. However, there are no other features of tuberous sclerosis, such as subependymal nodules or cortical tubers, although these would be difficult to visualise on CT unless they were calcified. A patient with tuberous sclerosis would also have a history of seizures.

FURTHER INVESTIGATIONS AND MANAGEMENT

1. MRI of brain, pre- and post-contrast images.
2. Neurosurgical referral.

FURTHER INFORMATION

Colloid cyst can often be hyperdense on pre-contrast CT and hyperintense on T1 MRI due to the presence of proteinaceous debris. There may be feint enhancement of the rim of the cyst. Colloid cysts can cause positional headache. A seemingly innocuous colloid cyst can cause acute hydrocephalus and sometimes lead to sudden death.

Subependymal giant-cell astrocytoma is seen mainly in patients with tuberous sclerosis. These tumours enhance on post-contrast images. The differential diagnoses of a third ventricular tumour include colloid cyst, giant-cell astrocytoma, central neurocytoma, metastasis, chordoid glioma and suprasellar extension of craniopharyngioma.

CASE 2.6: 50-YEAR-OLD MAN WITH CHEST PAIN

Figure v2.6a

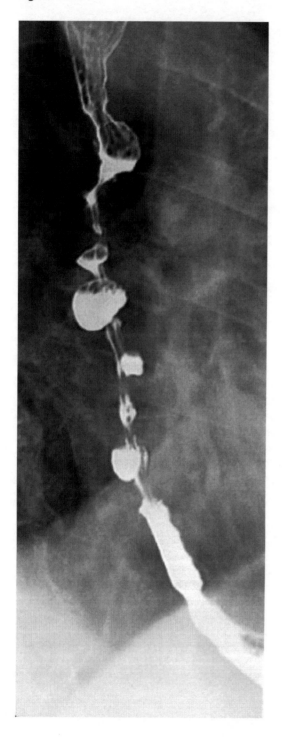

CORKSCREW OESOPHAGUS

FINDINGS

Double-contrast barium swallow, lateral projection:
1. Series of indentations of barium column along the oesophagus resembling a 'corkscrew'.

MAIN DIAGNOSIS

Given the history of chest pain, the appearance is consistent with diffuse oesophageal spasm.

DIFFERENTIAL DIAGNOSIS

Nutcracker oesophagus. However, the imaging findings are usually non-specific and the diagnosis is based on manometric studies.

FURTHER INVESTIGATIONS AND MANAGEMENT

1. Oesophageal manometry may be required.
2. Also check for gastro-oesophageal reflux, as there is an association.
3. Generally, medical management with nitrates and calcium-channel blockers.

FURTHER INFORMATION

Symptoms of diffuse oesophageal spasm often resemble those of angina, and nitrates and nifedipine may relieve symptoms. There is a series of tertiary contractions that are uncoordinated and non-peristaltic. Diffuse oesophageal spasm may be intermittent, and therefore 24-hour manometric studies may be necessary. At least 30% of swallows must be affected for the diagnosis to be made. There may be severe thickening of the oesophageal wall in diffuse oesophageal spasm. In nutcracker oesophagus, the contractions are primary peristaltic but the pressures are very high. On barium swallow, normal peristalsis is visualised and the diagnosis is based on manometry.

CASE 2.7: 50-YEAR-OLD WOMAN WITH LEG WEAKNESS

Figure v2.7a

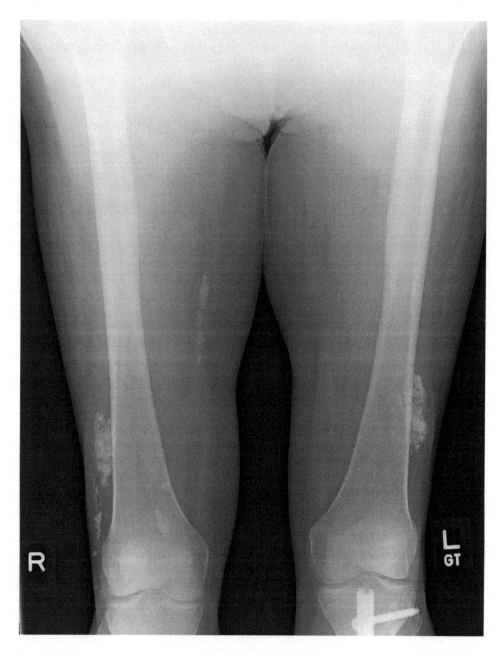

DERMATOMYOSITIS

FINDINGS

1. 'Sheet-like' symmetrical calcification of thigh soft tissue.
2. Apparent atrophy of the thigh muscles with linear low-density areas, possibly due to fatty infiltration.
3. Intramedullary nail within the left tibia.
4. Knee joints are normal.

MAIN DIAGNOSIS

Dermatomyositis.

DIFFERENTIAL DIAGNOSIS

Scleroderma. However, this is unlikely as soft tissue calcification in scleroderma occurs over large joints and pressure areas.

FURTHER INVESTIGATIONS AND MANAGEMENT

1. MRI is helpful for identifying the affected muscle groups.
2. As dermatomyositis is strongly associated with malignant disease, CT of thorax, abdomen and pelvis must be considered.
3. Creatine kinase measurement to assess the disease activity.
4. Electromyography to confirm the presence of myopathy.
5. Rheumatology referral.

FURTHER INFORMATION

Dermatomyositis is an autoimmune condition that affects striated muscles and skin. It causes inflammation and muscle atrophy, and finally calcification and fibrosis with flexion contractures and ulcerations. Chest X-ray can show bilateral pulmonary infiltrates or basal interstitial fibrosis, similar to scleroderma. Another chest X-ray pattern is aspiration pneumonia, due to pharyngeal muscle weakness and oesophageal atony. There is an increased incidence of malignancy, particularly of the ovaries, lung and gastrointestinal tract.

CASE 2.8: 45-YEAR-OLD WOMAN WITH BACK PAIN RADIATING TO LEFT LEG

Figures v2.8a, v2.8b (L4-5 level) and v2.8c (L4-5 level)

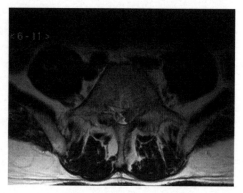

b

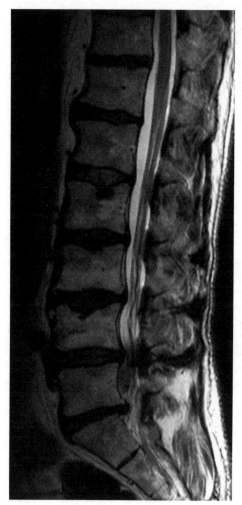

a

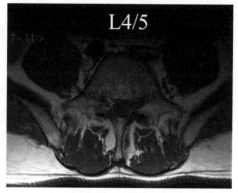

c

L4–5 INTERVERTEBRAL DISC EXTRUSION

FINDINGS

Lumbosacral spine MRI:
1. Low T2 and intermediate T1 signal material posterior to the L4–5 disc space and posterior and to the left of L5 vertebral body
2. The left L5 nerve root is compressed and displaced posteriorly at the left lateral recess
3. Circumferential disc bulge at L4–5
4. Mild L5–S1 disc protrusion
5. Schmorl's node at the superior endplate L2
6. L4 superior endplate compression fracture.

DIAGNOSIS

L4–5 left paracentral disc extrusion compressing the left L5 nerve root at the left lateral recess.

FURTHER MANAGEMENT

Urgent neurosurgical referral for potential intervertebral disc surgery.

FURTHER INFORMATION

In the cervical spine, there are seven vertebrae but eight nerve roots. The C1 nerve root exits above C1, and the C2 nerve root exits between C1 and C2. The C8 nerve root exits between C7 and T1. Within the thoracic spine, the T1 nerve root exits between T1 and T2 and the T12 nerve root exits between T12 and L1. Within the lumbar spine, the nerve roots exit below the pedicle of the same-numbered vertebra, well above the intervertebral disc space. Thus paracentral disc herniations in the lumbar spine can compress nerve roots that exit below the intervertebral disc space. For example, L2 paracentral disc protrusion can compress the L3 nerve root at the lateral recess.

CASE 2.9: NEONATE WITH VOMITING

Figure v2.9a

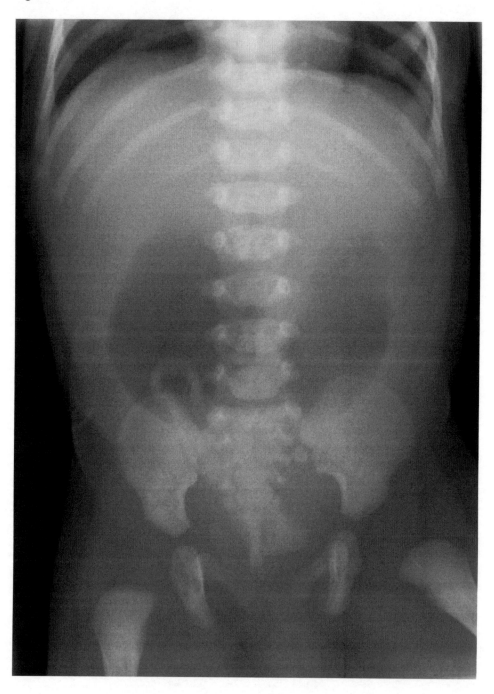

DUODENAL ATRESIA

FINDINGS

1. Midline 'double-bubble' sign, consistent with dilated gas-filled stomach and proximal duodenum.
2. Lack of gas elsewhere within the abdomen.

MAIN DIAGNOSIS

Duodenal atresia.

DIFFERENTIAL DIAGNOSIS

1. Duodenal stenosis.
2. Duodenal web.
3. Annular pancreas.
4. Malrotation and midgut volvulus.

All of the above diagnoses can present with a 'double-bubble' sign on abdominal radiograph. However, the complete absence of gas distal to the duodenum makes these possibilities less likely.

FURTHER INVESTIGATIONS AND MANAGEMENT

1. Urgent paediatric surgical referral. Complete or partial obstruction of the duodenum requires surgical treatment.
2. If there is any potential delay in surgery, abdominal ultrasound and upper GI contrast study may be required, in particular to exclude malrotation and midgut volvulus.

FURTHER INFORMATION

Duodenal atresia is a common cause of bilious vomiting in the first 24 hours after birth. Duodenal atresia, stenosis and web all result from incomplete recanalisation of the duodenum during the 10th gestational week. Obstruction is below the level of the ampulla of Vater, hence the bilious vomiting.

CASE 2.10: 49-YEAR-OLD MAN WITH SEVERE LEFT ILIAC FOSSA PAIN AND PERITONISM

Figures v2.10a and v2.10b

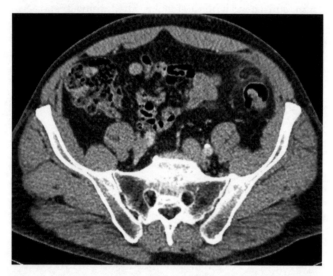

a

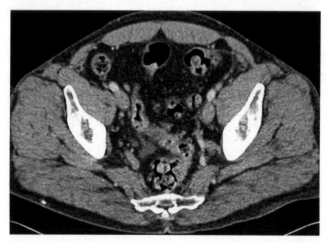

b

EPIPLOIC APPENDAGITIS

FINDINGS

1. Pericolonic oval low-attenuation structure in the left iliac fossa which has a slightly higher attenuation than normal fat, and which is surrounded by a hyperattenuating rim.
2. Inflammatory stranding of the surrounding fat.
3. Thickening of the adjacent parietal peritoneum.
4. Small amount of pelvic free fluid.

MAIN DIAGNOSIS

Epiploic appendagitis.

DIFFERENTIAL DIAGNOSIS

Segmental omental infarction. However, this usually occurs on the right side of the abdomen.

FURTHER INVESTIGATIONS AND MANAGEMENT

1. No further investigation is necessary.
2. Non-surgical treatment.

FURTHER INFORMATION

Epiploic appendages are elongated fatty structures that arise from the serosal surface of the colon. Clinically, epiploic appendagitis mimics diverticulitis or appendicitis. Epiploic appendages are supplied by the vasa recta of the colon. Torsion or venous thrombosis of an appendage causes acute infarction followed by localised inflammation.

CASE 2.11: 61-YEAR-OLD MAN WITH LONG-STANDING COGNITIVE DECLINE

Figures v2.11a, v2.11b and v2.11c

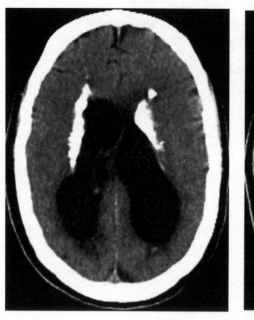

a

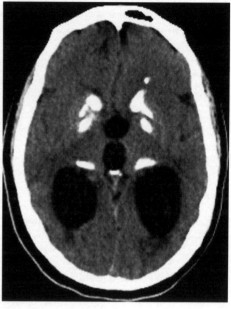

b

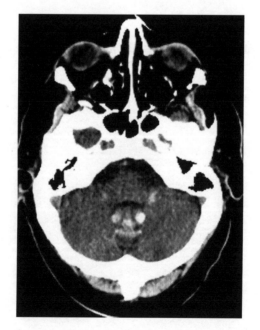

c

FAHR'S DISEASE

FINDINGS

1. Dense calcification of bilateral caudate and lentiform nuclei, thalami and dentate nuclei.
2. Predominantly central cerebral atrophy.
3. Periventricular low attenuation consistent with mild chronic small-vessel disease.

MAIN DIAGNOSIS

Fahr's disease.

DIFFERENTIAL DIAGNOSIS

1. Metabolic: hyperparathyroidism, hypoparathyroidism, MELAS.
2. Congenital: Down syndrome, Cockayne syndrome.
3. Post-inflammatory: congenital HIV, toxoplasmosis, TB.
4. Ischaemic: carbon monoxide poisoning, anoxia.

FURTHER INVESTIGATIONS AND MANAGEMENT

1. As this is a diagnosis of exclusion, other secondary causes of calcification of bilateral basal ganglia must be excluded first.
2. The symptoms show considerable similarities to those of Parkinson's disease. Therefore a full neurological assessment should be recommended.

FURTHER INFORMATION

There are several causes of calcification of basal ganglia, as outlined above. The other name for Fahr's disease is bilateral striatopallidodentate calcinosis (BSPDC). Clinical features include Parkinsonism, chorea, dystonia, ataxia and dementia.

CASE 2.12: 49-YEAR-OLD WOMAN WITH LEG SWELLING

Figure v2.12a

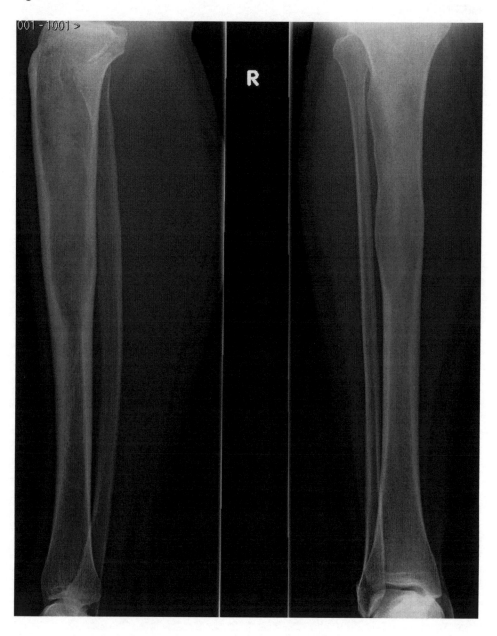

FIBROUS DYSPLASIA

FINDINGS

1. Expansile ground-glass-density lesion arising from the tibial upper diametaphyseal region.
2. The lesion is based within the medullary cavity and is longitudinally orientated.
3. Endosteal scalloping.
4. Narrow zone of transition with a cortical rind around the lesion.
5. No cortical destruction.
6. No soft tissue mass.

MAIN DIAGNOSIS

Fibrous dysplasia.

DIFFERENTIAL DIAGNOSIS

1. Enchondroma. However, this is unlikely as there is no chondroid-type matrix mineralisation.
2. Aneurysmal bone cyst. However, this is unlikely as it occurs in younger subjects.
3. Solitary bone cyst. However, this is unlikely as it, too, occurs in younger subjects. The upper tibia is also an unlikely location for this lesion.
4. Adamantinoma. This is a possibility, but it is a very rare tumour.

FURTHER INVESTIGATIONS AND MANAGEMENT

1. Orthopaedic referral.
2. Assessment for endocrine abnormalities.

FURTHER INFORMATION

In fibrous dysplasia, the normal medullary bone is replaced by fibrous tissue, cartilage and cystic areas containing haematogenous and serous fluid. The fibrous stroma can become ossified, giving rise to increased density. On plain radiographs, fibrous dysplasia appears as an expansile, bubbly lesion that is lucent to ground-glass density, with a narrow zone of transition. The lesions are diametaphyseal in location. There is no periosteal reaction and there is no soft tissue mass associated with the lesion. The ribs, long bones, pelvis and skull base may become affected. Fibrous dysplasia can be divided into two types, namely monostotic and polyostotic. McCune–Albright syndrome is a combination of polyostotic fibrous dysplasia, precocious puberty and skin pigmentation. Fibrous dysplasia appears as hot lesions on MDP bone scan.

CASE 2.13: 45-YEAR-OLD MAN WITH A 6-WEEK HISTORY OF DRY COUGH AND SHORTNESS OF BREATH

Figures v2.13a and v2.13b

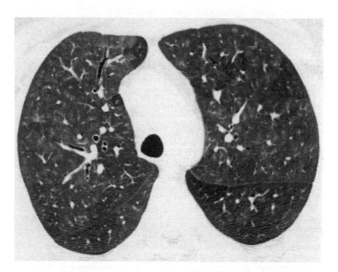

a

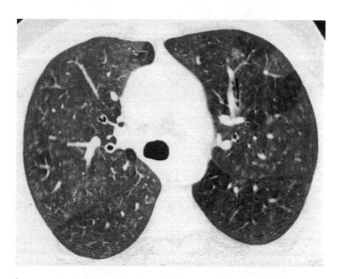

b

SUBACUTE HYPERSENSITIVITY PNEUMONITIS

FINDINGS

1. Patchy bilateral ground-glass opacification.
2. Small ill-defined centrilobular nodules with ground-glass attenuation.
3. Focal areas of decreased attenuation corresponding to secondary pulmonary lobules anteriorly within the upper lobes and apical segment of the left lower lobe, giving rise to mosaic perfusion.

MAIN DIAGNOSIS

Subacute hypersensitivity pneumonitis (extrinsic allergic alveolitis).

DIFFERENTIAL DIAGNOSIS

Respiratory bronchiolitis associated with interstitial lung disease (RB-ILD). This is associated with cigarette smoking, and there is often bronchial wall thickening in addition to ground-glass changes and centrilobular nodules.

FURTHER INVESTIGATIONS AND MANAGEMENT

1. Occupational and social history.
2. Enquire whether there are any pets in the patient's home.
3. History of smoking.

FURTHER INFORMATION

Hypersensitivity pneumonitis is caused by inhalation of organic particles or fumes. The subacute form is caused by continuous exposure to low doses of organic dusts or fumes, whereas the acute form is caused by exposure to large doses of antigen. Chronic disease is also caused by exposure to low doses of antigen over a long period of time, leading to pulmonary fibrosis. Patchy ground-glass opacification, mosaic attenuation due to air trapping and centrilobular nodules are HRCT features of subacute hypersensitivity pneumonitis. The features of subacute hypersensitivity pneumonitis are very similar to those of RB-ILD, which is associated with cigarette smoking. Patchy ground-glass opacification, centrilobular nodularity and bronchial wall thickening are the three main HRCT features of RB-ILD. The findings of RB-ILD are predominantly in the upper lobes, and there is often upper zone emphysema.

CASE 2.14: 81-YEAR-OLD MAN WITH NEUTROPENIA

Figures v2.14a and v2.14b

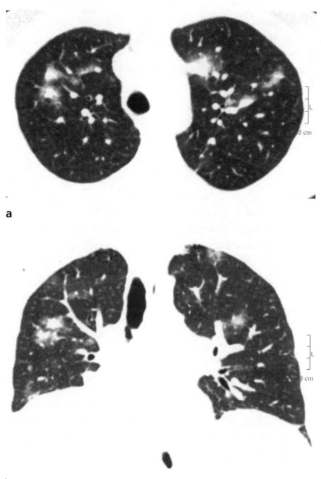

a

b

INVASIVE PULMONARY ASPERGILLOSIS

FINDINGS

1. Multiple bilateral, randomly scattered, dense pulmonary nodules.
2. Halo of ground glass surrounding the nodules (the CT halo sign).

MAIN DIAGNOSIS

Invasive pulmonary aspergillosis.

DIFFERENTIAL DIAGNOSIS

Multiple pulmonary nodules with apparent CT halo sign. The differential diagnosis is wide, as the CT halo sign can be present in the following conditions:
1. Infections: candida, CMV, TB, coccidioidomycosis, legionella.
2. Non-infectious conditions: Wegener's granulomatosis, bronchoalveolar cell carcinoma, adenocarcinoma, sarcoidosis, metastatic angiosarcoma and Kaposi's sarcoma.

FURTHER INVESTIGATIONS AND MANAGEMENT

1. Sputum microscopy and culture.
2. Serum precipitins.
3. Urgent medical referral for early antifungal treatment.

FURTHER INFORMATION

Angioinvasive aspergillosis causes infiltration of lung tissues and invasion of small blood vessels. In neutropenic patients, the presence of nodules with the CT halo sign is sufficient to allow a presumptive diagnosis of invasive aspergillosis. The halo in the CT halo sign is secondary to a ring of coagulation necrosis and haemorrhage. The central dense nodule is produced by a central fungal nodule or infarction. As the lesions heal, these nodules often cavitate, and characteristic air crescents develop.

CASE 2.15: 54-YEAR-OLD MAN WITH CHEST PAIN

Figure v2.15a

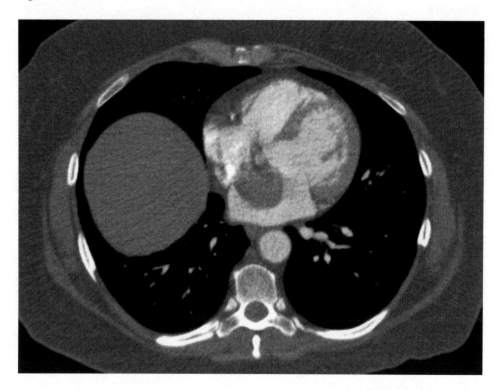

LEFT ATRIAL MYXOMA

FINDINGS

1. Low-attenuation filling defect within the left atrium, which appears to be attached to the inter-atrial septum.
2. No calcification of the mass.
3. Attenuation of the mass higher than that of fatty tissues.

MAIN DIAGNOSIS

Left atrial myxoma.

DIFFERENTIAL DIAGNOSIS

1. Left atrial thrombus.
2. Metastasis.
3. Sarcoma.
4. Fibroelastoma.

FURTHER INVESTIGATIONS AND MANAGEMENT

1. Cardiac MRI for better identification of the stalk.
2. Urgent cardiothoracic referral with a view to surgical excision.
3. Look for signs of sexual precocity, hyperpigmented skin lesions and Cushing's syndrome, as cardiac myxomas can be associated with Carney complex.

FURTHER INFORMATION

Myxoma is the most common benign cardiac tumour. Myxomas most frequently arise from the left atrium, and are attached by a thin stalk at the fossa ovalis. Patients may present with fever, weight loss and arthralgia, and clinical findings include clubbing and positional murmur. Left atrial myxoma can cause pulmonary venous hypertension and pulmonary oedema. Angiosarcoma is the most common malignant cardiac tumour.

CASE 2.16: 23-YEAR-OLD WOMAN WITH BILATERAL GROIN PAIN

Figure v2.16a

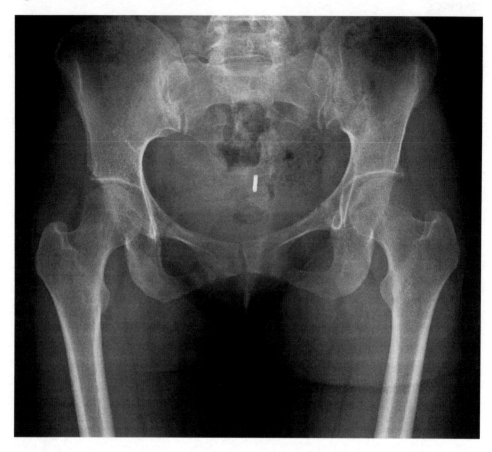

OSTEOMALACIA

FINDINGS

1. Slight generalised reduction in bone density.
2. Bilateral symmetrical ill-defined radiolucent lines perpendicular to the bony cortex, affecting both superior and inferior pubic rami.
3. Some marginal sclerosis but no callus formation.
4. No displacement.
5. Normal proximal femora.

DIAGNOSIS

Looser's zones or pseudofractures, consistent with osteomalacia.

FURTHER INVESTIGATIONS AND MANAGEMENT

1. Medical referral.
2. Check vitamin D, calcium, phosphate and alkaline phosphatase levels, and renal function.

FURTHER INFORMATION

Osteomalacia results from vitamin D deficiency in the mature skeleton. Looser's zones are subclinical insufficiency fractures that are repaired by unossified bone. Typical locations include the scapulae, medial femoral necks, ischio-pubic rami, lower ribs and ulna. In developing countries, osteomalacia is secondary to dietary deficiency of vitamin D, calcium or phosphorus. In the developed world, vitamin D deficiency is due to malabsorption or renal disease. Other skeletal manifestations of osteomalacia include bowing of long bones, protrusio acetabuli, and biconcave vertebral body fractures.

CASE 2.17: JAW PAIN

Figure v2.17a

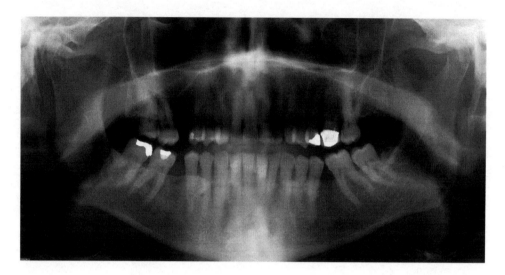

MYELOMA OF THE JAW

FINDINGS

1. Orthopantomogram shows well-defined lytic lesions at the right mandibular condyle and left angle of the mandible.
2. There is also a minimally displaced pathological fracture through the right condylar neck.

MAIN DIAGNOSIS

Multiple myeloma affecting the jaw, with a pathological fracture through the right condylar neck.

DIFFERENTIAL DIAGNOSIS

1. Multiple bone metastases. However, in the mandible, myeloma is more common than metastases.
2. Eosinophilic granuloma, especially if the patient is young.
3. Brown tumours of hyperparathyroidism. However, there is no evidence of loss of the lamina dura. There are high calcium, low phosphate and high parathormone levels in patients with hyperparathyroidism.

FURTHER INVESTIGATIONS AND MANAGEMENT

1. Explore the history of malignancy, particularly of lung, breast and kidney.
2. Skeletal survey and biochemical profile.
3. Medical referral.

FURTHER INFORMATION

Diffuse osteoporosis and focal lytic lesions are the two most important radiological features of multiple myeloma. Lytic foci are located in the long bones, axial skeleton and skull. Lesions appear as irregular punched-out lysis with endosteal scalloping. Myeloma may also involve the mandible and clavicles, both of which are sites that are rarely affected by metastases.

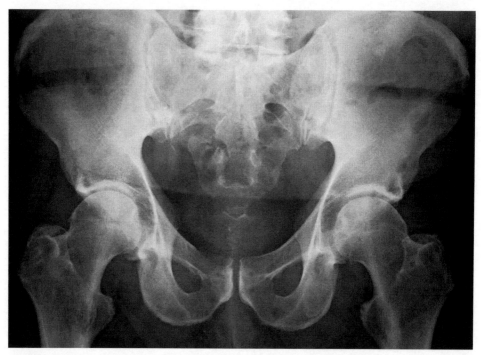

Figure v2.17b: Further examples of multiple myeloma. X-ray of the pelvis showing lesions of the pubic rami with pathological fracture of the right superior pubic ramus.

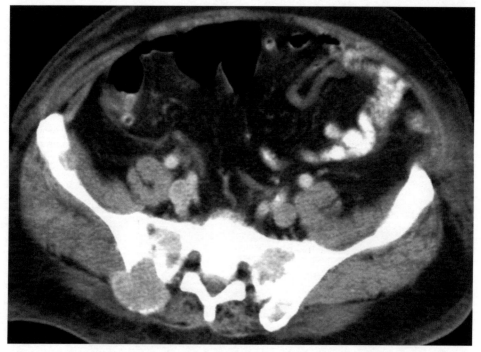

Figure v2.17c: CT of the pelvis showing lytic masses with soft tissue component.

CASE 2.18: NEONATE WITH RESPIRATORY DISTRESS

Figure v2.18a

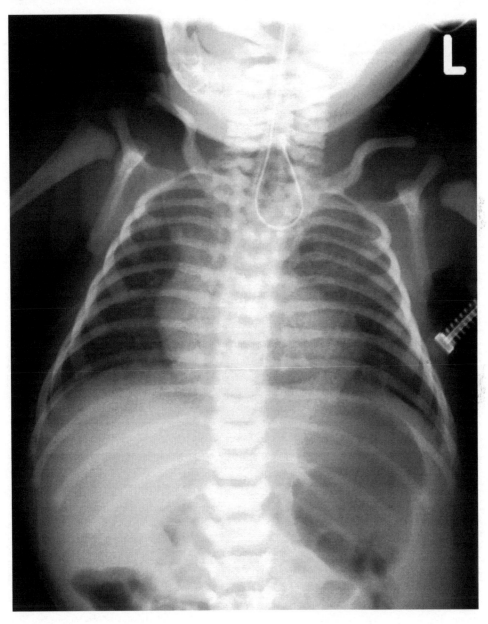

OESOPHAGEAL ATRESIA

FINDINGS

1. A coiled nasogastric tube within a dilated upper oesophagus at the thoracic inlet.
2. Gas present within the stomach.
3. 13 pairs of ribs.
4. No vertebral body segmentation anomalies.

DIAGNOSIS

Oesophageal atresia with coexisting distal tracheo-oesophageal fistula.

FURTHER INVESTIGATIONS AND MANAGEMENT

1. Urgent surgical referral.
2. US abdomen and echocardiography scan to assess renal and cardiac anomalies.

FURTHER INFORMATION

There is a strong association between oesophageal atresia and other VACTERL anomalies. Oesophageal atresia is also associated with Down syndrome. A tracheo-oesophageal fistula may or may not be present. Oesophageal atresia with a distal tracheo-oesophageal fistula is the most common type of oesophageal atresia.

CASE 2.19: INFANT WITH FAILURE TO THRIVE

Figure v2.19a

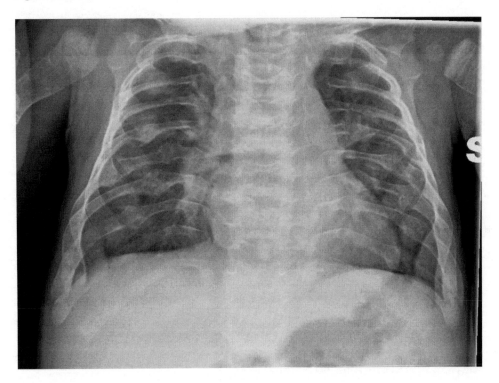

OSTEOGENESIS IMPERFECTA

FINDINGS

1. Generalised osteopenia, loss of normal trabeculation and cortical thinning.
2. Gracile bones.
3. Multiple bilateral rib fractures with callus formation.
4. Biconcave vertebral body fractures.
5. Sclerotic humeral metaphyseal lines, most probably due to pamidronate treatment.
6. Lungs clear.

MAIN DIAGNOSIS

Osteogenesis imperfecta. The patient is most probably on bisphosphonate treatment, as evidenced by the dense metaphyseal lines.

DIFFERENTIAL DIAGNOSIS

1. Rickets. However, there is no evidence of cupping and fraying of the metaphyses. Beading in rickets occurs at the costochondral junction.
2. Non-accidental injury. However, this is less likely as the rib fractures are both anterior and posterior and there are no metaphyseal corner or bucket-handle fractures.

FURTHER INVESTIGATIONS AND MANAGEMENT

1. History of fractures of other bones, and examination for presence of blue sclerae.
2. Family history.
3. Medical referral for further management.

FURTHER INFORMATION

Osteogenesis imperfecta is secondary to defective collagen, leading to abnormalities of bones, joints, skin and sclera. There are four main types of osteogenesis imperfecta:
- Type I: the most common type, the main features of which are mild bone fragility, blue sclera and deafness.
- Type II: lethal *in utero* or in early infancy.
- Type III: severe form, the main features of which are blue sclerae, osteoporotic bones, multiple fractures, kyphoscoliosis and wormian bones.
- Type IV: mild bone fragility and normal sclera.

CASE 2.20: 65-YEAR-OLD MAN WITH EPIGASTRIC PAIN

Figure v2.20a

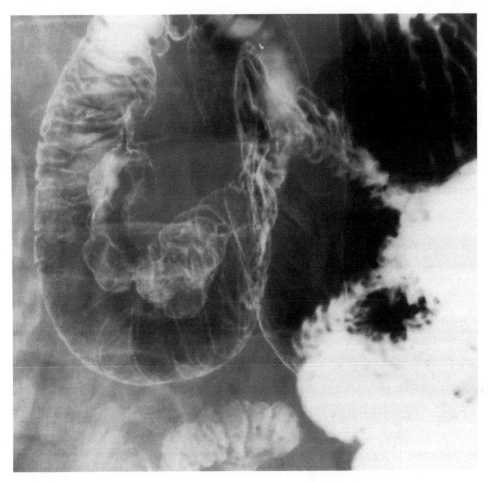

PANCREATIC CARCINOMA

FINDINGS

Barium meal examination:
1. Large irregular lobulated filling defect arising from the medial wall of the second part of the duodenum
2. Distortion of the medial wall of the second part of the duodenum in 'reverse 3' pattern.

MAIN DIAGNOSIS

Carcinoma of the head of the pancreas invading the duodenum.

DIFFERENTIAL DIAGNOSIS

1. Carcinoma of the ampulla of Vater.
2. Periampullary duodenal carcinoma.

Both of these conditions can appear as an irregular filling defect within the duodenum, and cannot be distinguished on the basis of the barium study alone.

FURTHER INVESTIGATIONS AND MANAGEMENT

1. CT chest, abdomen and pelvis for staging, including dual-phase (arterial and portovenous) CT through the pancreas.
2. Endoscopic biopsy with or without ERCP for biliary stenting.

FURTHER INFORMATION

Pancreatic masses are currently investigated with dual-phase CT. Occasionally these may be discovered in a barium meal examination that has been performed for other indications. Carcinoma of the head of the pancreas affects the inner margin of the duodenal loop and the adjacent pylorus. Large masses can splay the duodenal loop, and if there is invasion of the duodenum there is often irregularity and architectural distortion of the duodenum. The 'reverse 3' sign is due to indentation of the duodenum by the pancreatic mass. Chronic pancreatitis can also cause indentation of the duodenum, giving rise to a similar appearance.

CASE 2.21: 2-YEAR-OLD BOY WITH GROWTH RETARDATION

Figure v2.21a

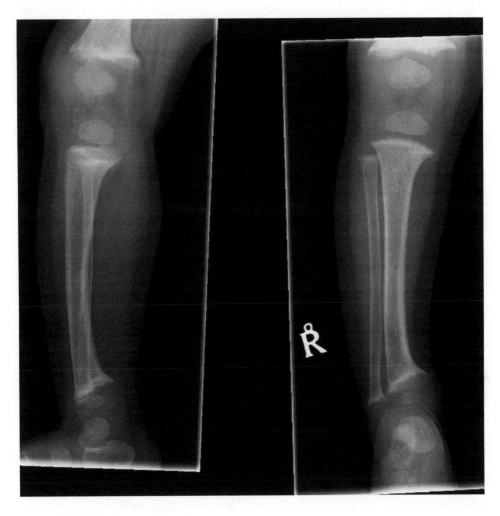

RICKETS

FINDINGS

Right lower leg radiograph:
1. Generalised osteopenia
2. Bowing of the tibia
3. Widening of the physis
4. Metaphyseal cupping and fraying
5. Thin metaphyseal spurs.

MAIN DIAGNOSIS

Rickets.

DIFFERENTIAL DIAGNOSIS

1. Renal tubular acidosis. This is radiographically indistinguishable from vitamin D deficiency rickets.
2. Osteogenesis imperfecta. A family history may be present. The child may also have blue sclerae.

FURTHER INVESTIGATIONS AND MANAGEMENT

Medical referral for further work-up regarding the cause of rickets.

FURTHER INFORMATION

The aetiology of rickets can broadly be divided into two categories:
*   vitamin D deficiency rickets (parathormone levels are elevated)
*   phosphate deficiency rickets (normal parathormone levels).

In addition to the findings described above, other skeletal changes of rickets include triradiate pelvis, Harrison's sulcus, biconcave vertebral bodies, basilar invagination and craniotabes. There may also be pathological fractures and periosteal reaction.

CASE 2.22: 16-YEAR-OLD GIRL WITH COUGH

Figure v2.22a

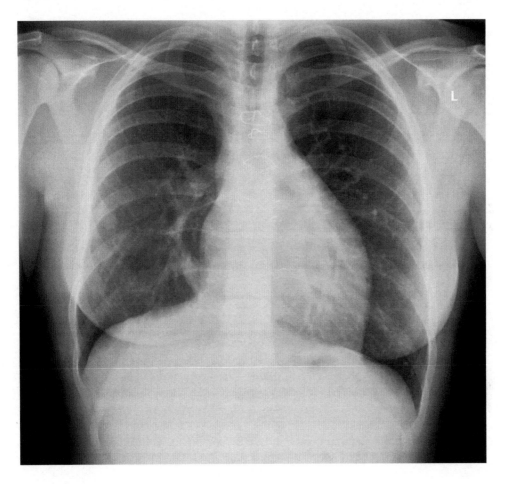

SCIMITAR SYNDROME

FINDINGS

1. Central sternotomy wires.
2. A curved tubular opacity parallels the right heart border, extending inferomedially from the right hilum to the right cardiophrenic angle.
3. Mildly reduced volume of the right hemithorax.
4. Normal left-sided position of the cardiac apex.

DIAGNOSIS

Scimitar syndrome (or pulmonary venolobar syndrome). The presence of the sternotomy wires suggests that there has been previous corrective surgery for a left to right shunt.

FURTHER INVESTIGATIONS AND MANAGEMENT

1. Review previous films.
2. Establish the nature of previous cardiac surgery.

FURTHER INFORMATION

Scimitar syndrome is also called pulmonary venolobar syndrome or hypogenetic lung syndrome. It affects the right lung, and in the complete form there is ipsilateral partial anomalous pulmonary venous return to the sub- or supra-diaphragmatic portion of the inferior vena cava, right lung hypoplasia, dextrorotation of the heart and anomalous arterial supply to the right lower lobe from the thoracic aorta. The anomalous vein can sometimes drain directly into the right atrium, coronary sinus, or portal or hepatic veins. Scimitar syndrome can be associated with congenital heart disease, most commonly atrial septal defect. CTPA or MR angiography can be used for confirmation and anatomical outline of the anomalous vein and any coexisting pulmonary and cardiac anomalies.

Viva 3

CASE 3.1: 70-YEAR-OLD BEING INVESTIGATED FOR ANAEMIA

Figure v3.1a

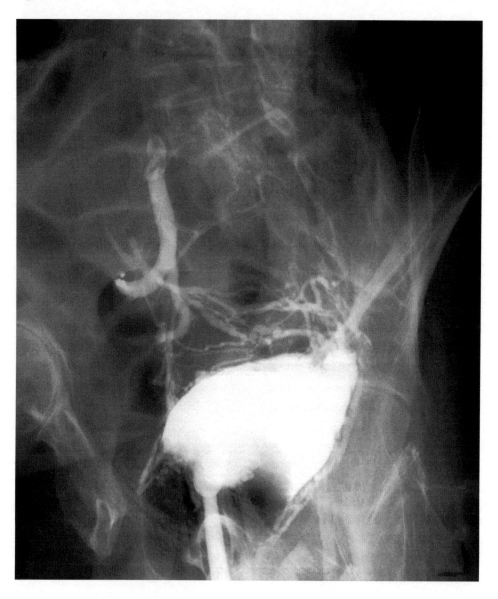

BARIUM VENOUS INTRAVASATION

FINDINGS

1. Barium enema examination: view of the rectum.
2. Rectal catheter *in situ*.
3. Barium visualised within the perirectal and larger draining veins.

DIAGNOSIS

Venous intravasation of barium.

FURTHER INVESTIGATIONS AND MANAGEMENT

1. Immediately stop the examination, deflate the balloon and remove the catheter.
2. Watch for cardiopulmonary symptoms and signs secondary to barium pulmonary embolism.
3. 'Head-up' position of the enema table with the patient turned to the right has been recommended to retard passage of barium into the pulmonary circulation.
4. Immediate communication with the clinical team, as the patient will require admission for close cardiopulmonary, hepatic, renal and coagulopathy monitoring.

FURTHER INFORMATION

Venous intravasation of barium is a rare but serious complication of barium enema examination. The mortality rate for barium pulmonary embolism is up to 80%. High rectal venous intravasation results in barium embolism into the portal venous system, and the mortality rate is lower than that of low rectal venous intravasation, which can lead to pulmonary embolism. Venous intravasation of barium is more likely to occur in elderly patients with colorectal disease, and in elderly female patients in whom a rectal catheter has been inadvertently placed into the vagina.

CASE 3.2: PAINFUL HIP AND LOW-GRADE FEVER

Figure v3.2a

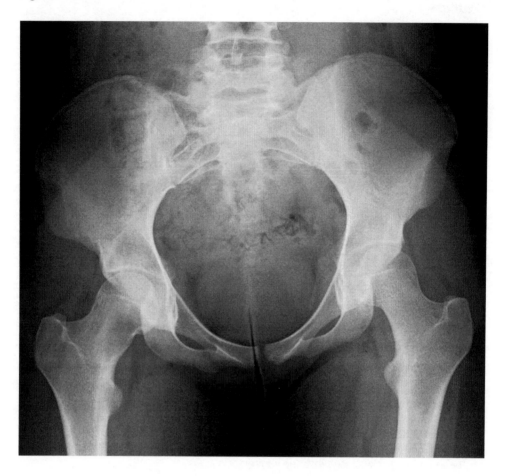

BRODIE'S ABSCESS

FINDINGS

1. Lytic expansile lesion along the medial border of the right femoral neck.
2. Metaphyseal location.
3. Well-defined broad sclerotic border with narrow zone of transition suggestive of a benign lesion.
4. Young patient – note the unfused iliac crest epiphyses.

MAIN DIAGNOSIS

Brodie's abscess.

DIFFERENTIAL DIAGNOSIS

1. Non-ossifying fibroma. However, this is unlikely as these do not tend to be symptomatic.
2. Healing eosinophilic granuloma or brown tumour. There may also be lesions present elsewhere.
3. Fibrous dysplasia. However, this is unlikely as there is no ground-glass matrix.

FURTHER INVESTIGATIONS AND MANAGEMENT

1. Orthopaedic referral for blood culture and antibiotic treatment.
2. MRI for further evaluation may be necessary.

FURTHER INFORMATION

Brodie's abscess is a localised form of chronic osteomyelitis that is located in the metaphyseal regions of long bones. There is localised bone destruction with a narrow zone of transition. There may be surrounding sclerosis and periosteal reaction. Sometimes a finger-like extension towards the epiphyseal plate, known as 'tunnelling', may be present. A sequestrum, which is a piece of dead bone, may sometimes be present within the abscess. If there is a large amount of surrounding sclerosis, the radiographic findings may mimic osteoid osteoma.

CASE 3.3: 35-YEAR-OLD WOMAN WITH SHORTNESS OF BREATH

Figures v3.3a, v3.3b, v3.3c, v3.3d and v3.3e

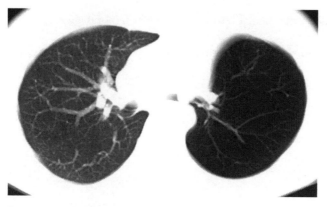

a

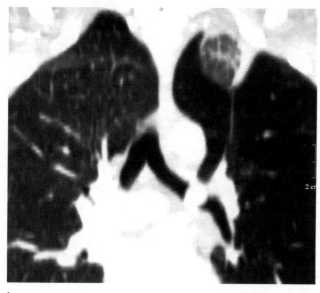

b

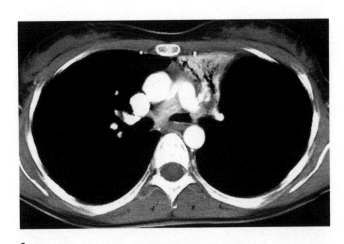

c

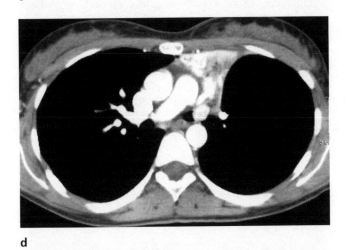

d

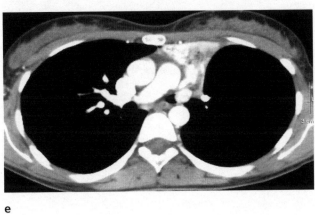

e

BRONCHIAL ADENOMA

FINDINGS

1. Small high-attenuation soft tissue density rounded nodule within the left main bronchus at the level of origin of the left upper lobe bronchus. No macroscopic calcification.
2. Complete occlusion of the left upper lobe bronchus causing left upper lobe collapse.
3. Partial obstruction of the left lower lobe bronchus causing air trapping, resulting in hyperlucent left lower lobe.

MAIN DIAGNOSIS

Bronchial adenoma, most probably bronchial carcinoid.

DIFFERENTIAL DIAGNOSIS

Endobronchial foreign body. However, there would be a history of foreign body aspiration.

FURTHER INVESTIGATIONS AND MANAGEMENT

1. Bronchoscopy.
2. Check for local lymph node and distant metastases, particularly to liver, adrenals and bone.
3. Surgical referral for resection.

FURTHER INFORMATION

Bronchial adenomas comprise a group of low-grade malignant tumours:
1. carcinoid (75%)
2. cylindroma
3. adenocystic carcinoma
4. mucoepidermoid carcinoma.

These tumours grow slowly but can metastasise to mediastinal lymph nodes and extra-thoracic sites such as liver, adrenals and bone. Pulmonary carcinoids are highly vascular tumours and are often calcified. Carcinoid syndrome is rare with pulmonary carcinoids.

CASE 3.4: 25-YEAR-OLD MAN WITH HIGH BLOOD PRESSURE

Figure v3.4a

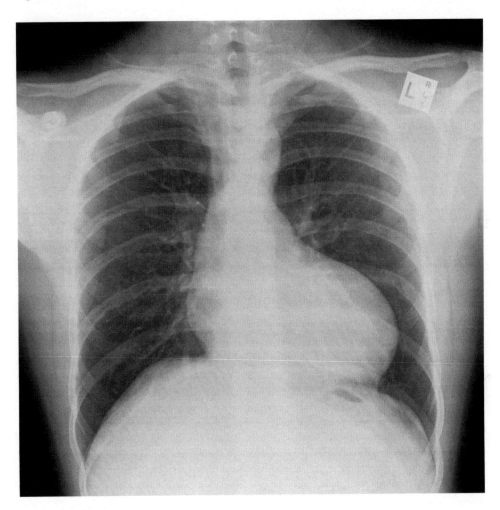

COARCTATION OF AORTA

FINDINGS

1. High position of the aortic arch with 'figure of 3' sign.
2. Bilateral inferior rib notching.
3. Cardiomegaly with rounding of the left heart border, consistent with left ventricular enlargement.
4. The lungs are clear.

MAIN DIAGNOSIS

Coarctation of aorta.

DIFFERENTIAL DIAGNOSIS

Aortic stenosis. However, this is unlikely given the history of hypertension and the presence of arch irregularity and rib notching.

FURTHER INVESTIGATIONS AND MANAGEMENT

1. Cardiology referral for consideration of stenting.
2. Echocardiogram.
3. Cardiac MRI and CT or MR angiography to assess the degree of stenosis and collateral formation.

FURTHER INFORMATION

Coarctation is usually at the level of the ligamentum arteriosum, beyond the origin of the left subclavian artery. Severe coarctation of the aorta presents within the first few days to weeks after birth with cardiac failure. Less severe forms can present in later life with hypertension within the upper half of the body and hypotension in the lower half. The first and second intercostal arteries arise from the subclavian arteries, while the rest of the intercostals arise directly from the descending aorta. Rib notching is due to collateral filling of the intercostal arteries via the internal mammary arteries, and is therefore visualised in the third to ninth ribs. Presentation in adults does not tend to be associated with cardiac anomalies, in contrast to presentation in infants, which is associated with coexisting bicuspid aortic valve/ PDA/VSD/ASD/aortic stenosis or incompetence.

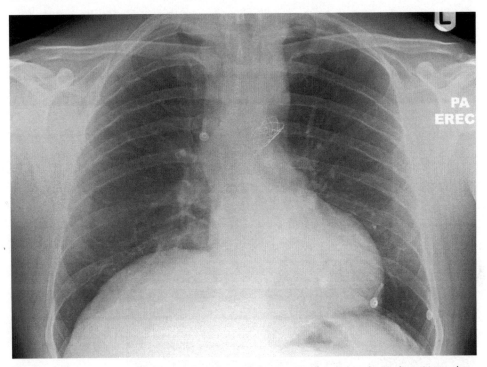

Figure v3.4b: Another case of coarctation of the aorta after stent insertion. Note the rib notching.

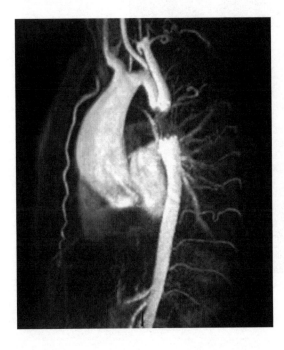

Figure v3.4c: MRI following stenting of the coarct segment. Signal drop-out produced by metal stent precludes accurate assessment of the luminal diameter at the level of the coarctation. There is aortic root dilatation. Distended internal mammary and intercostal arteries tend to suggest significant residual shunting. The true gradient across the coarctation can be assessed by interventional angiography.

CASE 3.5: 6-MONTH-OLD GIRL BEING INVESTIGATED FOR FIRST UTI

Figures v3.5a, v3.5b, v3.5c, v3.5d, v3.5e and v3.5f

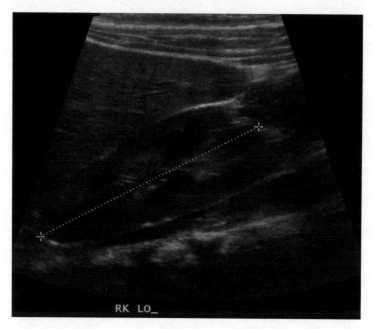

a

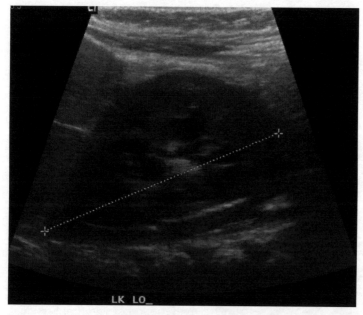

b

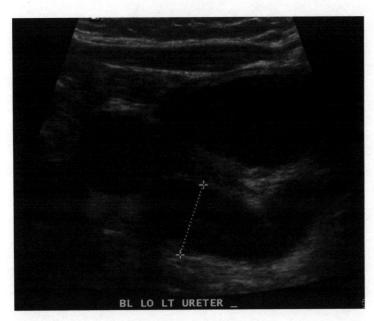

c

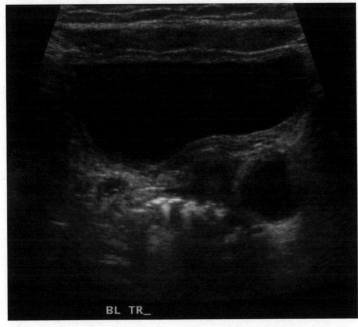

d

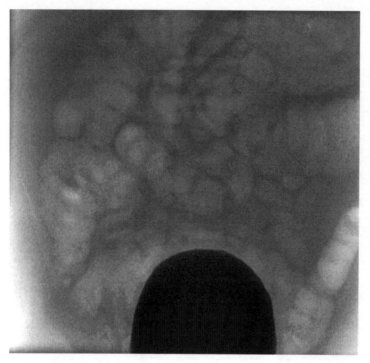

e

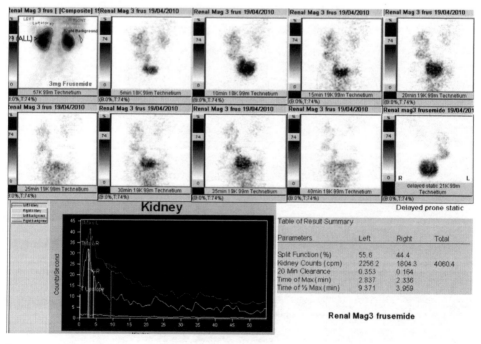

f

CONGENITAL (PRIMARY) MEGAURETER

FINDINGS

1. Renal ultrasound:
   a. Both kidneys are normal in size and appearance
   b. Left ureter dilated up to 13 mm, but no associated hydronephrosis
   c. Normal bladder
   d. No ureterocoele.
2. Micturating cystourethrogram (MCUG):
   a. No contrast reflux into the ureters.
3. MAG3 renogram:
   a. Split renal function (56% left and 44% right)
   b. Both kidneys have normal isotope uptake and excretion curves
   c. Left hydroureter.

INTERPRETATION

Dilated left ureter with normal drainage through the left kidney with no vesico-ureteric reflux.

MAIN DIAGNOSIS

Congenital (primary) left megaureter.

DIFFERENTIAL DIAGNOSIS

Megaureter secondary to urethral valves, neuropathic bladder, etc. However, this is unlikely as there is no evidence of vesico-ureteric reflux.

FURTHER INFORMATION

Congenital (primary) megaureter is due to abnormal musculature of the distal ureter causing focal lack of ureteric peristalsis (somewhat similar to achalasia and Hirschsprung's disease). It may be obstructed, non-obstructed, refluxing or non-obstructed non-refluxing. This case is of the non-obstructed non-refluxing type, which is the commonest type of neonatal (primary) megaureter. Primary megaureter is usually asymptomatic but can present with infection, haematuria or an abdominal mass, and may be associated with contralateral renal anomalies (e.g. renal agenesis, ectopia, PUJ obstruction, reflux, ureterocoele).

99m-Tc mercaptoacetyltriglycine (MAG3) renogram is a dynamic study. The steeply rising part of the curve shows the uptake proportional to the renal blood flow, the first 2–3 minutes thereafter is the measure of transit, and the rest of the curve indicates the excretory function. Unobstructed but dilated pelvis can be distinguished by its response to frusemide. If the renal activity decreases by more than 50% within 20 minutes of frusemide injection, obstruction is very unlikely, but if the activity remains constant or continues to rise, obstruction is highly likely.

99m-Tc dimercaptosuccinic acid (DMSA) is a static study and is used for imaging of functional renal cortical mass. Clinical applications include divided renal function, identification of functional renal tissue, differentiation of renal tissue from other adjacent masses, and assessment for renal scars.

CASE 3.6: 1-YEAR-OLD GIRL WITH HYDROCEPHALUS

Figures v3.6a, v3.6b, v3.6c and v3.6d

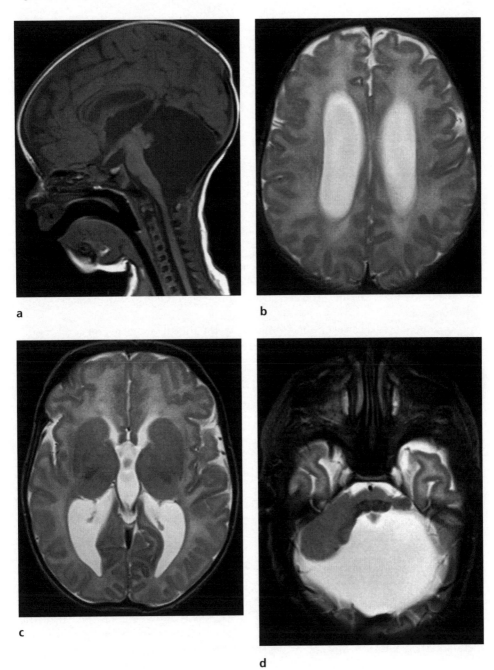

a

b

c

d

DANDY–WALKER MALFORMATION

FINDINGS

T1 sagittal and T2 axial MRI brain images:
1. The posterior fossa is enlarged, CSF filled and directly continuous with the fourth ventricle
2. Elevated tentorium cerebelli
3. Dysgenesis of cerebellar vermis
4. Small dysplastic and widely spaced cerebellar lobes
5. Thinning of the corpus callosum
6. Hydrocephalus.

MAIN DIAGNOSIS

Dandy–Walker malformation.

DIFFERENTIAL DIAGNOSIS

1. Mega cistern magna. However, this is unlikely as the cerebellar vermis and fourth ventricle would be expected to be normal in this condition.
2. Dandy–Walker variant. However, this is unlikely as the posterior fossa is enlarged.
3. Arachnoid cyst. However, this is unlikely as the fourth ventricle and cerebellar hemispheres would be expected to be normal but displaced.

FURTHER INVESTIGATIONS AND MANAGEMENT

Referral to neurosurgical team for consideration of CSF shunting.

FURTHER INFORMATION

Dandy–Walker syndrome is a congenital malformation that has three characteristic features:
1. agenesis/dysplasia of the cerebellar vermis
2. cystic dilatation of the fourth ventricle
3. enlarged posterior fossa.

The common associations include agenesis of the corpus callosum, lipoma of the corpus callosum, dysplasia of the cingulate gyrus, heterotopia and occipital encephalocoele. Dandy–Walker variant is a far more common presentation, in which the posterior fossa is of normal size. Arachnoid cyst should be considered in the differential diagnosis. This is typically retrocerebellar with associated mass effect on the cerebellum and fourth ventricle, and should not be confused with Dandy–Walker syndrome.

CASE 3.7: 30-YEAR-OLD WOMAN WITH KNEE PAIN

Figures v3.7a and v3.7b

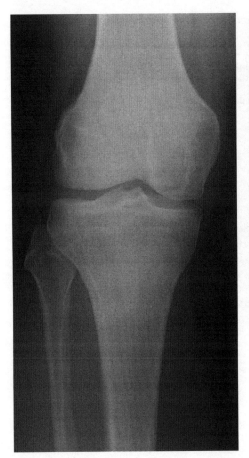

a

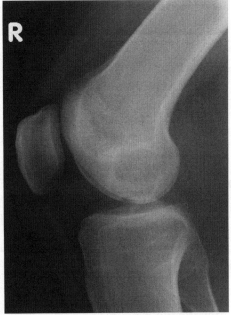

b

GIANT CELL TUMOUR

FINDINGS

1. Subarticular lucent lesion within the medial femoral condyle of a skeletally mature patient.
2. The lesion is eccentrically located.
3. Narrow zone of transition with well-defined sclerotic margins.
4. No internal mineralisation.
5. No periosteal reaction and no soft tissue mass.

MAIN DIAGNOSIS

Giant cell tumour.

DIFFERENTIAL DIAGNOSIS

1. Brodie's abscess. However, this is unlikely as it tends to be in the metaphyseal region. There is also no evidence of a sequestrum or periosteal reaction.
2. Metastasis. This is unlikely as the patient is young.
3. Geode. This is unlikely as there are no other features of degenerative disease of the joint.

FURTHER INVESTIGATIONS AND MANAGEMENT

1. As the presence of sclerotic margin is a rare occurrence in giant cell tumour, further evaluation with MRI has to be considered.
2. Orthopaedic referral with a view to curettage/resection.

FURTHER INFORMATION

Giant cell tumours have a characteristic appearance on plain radiographs, and arise from epiphyses or apophyses. These are well-defined eccentric lucent lesions which are sub-articular in location in patients after closure of epiphyses. The margins are well defined but mostly non-sclerotic. Chondroblastoma has a similar radiographic appearance in patients prior to closure of epiphyses. MRI may sometimes be necessary if there is diagnostic uncertainty. Giant cell tumour is low signal on T1 and mixed signal on T2 due to the presence of blood products and collagen matrix.

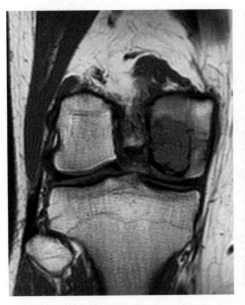

c

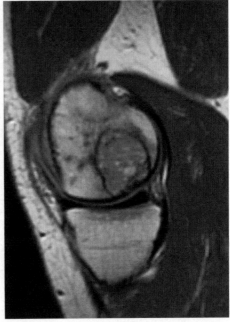

d

Figures v3.7c, v3.7d and v3.7e: T1 coronal and sagittal images showing low-signal subarticular lesion within the medial femoral condyle. Gradient echo sagittal image shows heterogeneous signal of the lesion with low-signal foci within it, most probably from haemosiderin deposits.

e

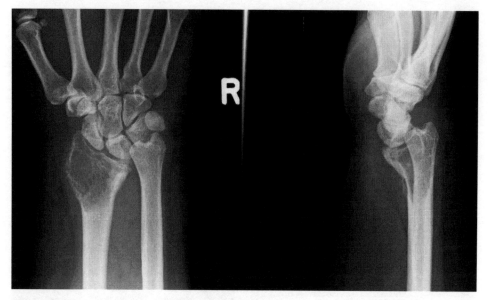

Figure v3.7f: An example of classical giant cell tumour – an eccentric, subarticular lesion with non-sclerotic relatively well-defined margins. Note the modelling deformity of the distal radius.

CASE 3.8: NEWBORN WITH FAILURE TO PASS MECONIUM

Figures v3.8a and v3.8b

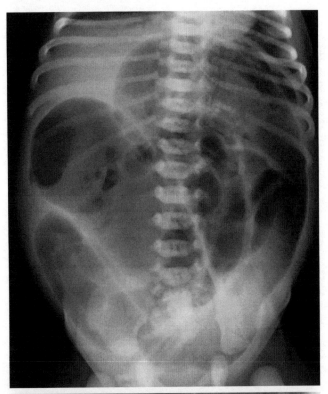

a

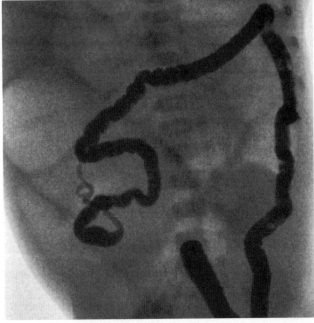

b

ILEAL ATRESIA

FINDINGS

1. Abdominal X-ray:
   a. Nasogastric tube *in situ*
   b. Markedly distended bowel loops
   c. No evidence of mottled lucencies in the right iliac fossa
   d. No free gas.
2. Water-soluble contrast enema:
   a. The entire colon is small in calibre
   b. Contrast refluxes into a small-calibre terminal ileum that ends abruptly.

MAIN DIAGNOSIS

Distal ileal atresia.

DIFFERENTIAL DIAGNOSIS

Meconium ileus. However, this is unlikely as there is no evidence of dilated distal ileum and caecum filled with pellets of meconium ('deer droppings').

FURTHER INVESTIGATIONS AND MANAGEMENT

Immediate paediatric surgery referral for resection of the atretic segment and bowel anastomosis.

FURTHER INFORMATION

Failure to pass meconium within the first 48 hours after birth, associated with distended bowel loops on abdominal radiograph, raises a number of possibilities. These are as follows (contrast enema findings are also provided).
1. Meconium ileus: microcolon, pellets of viscid meconium in the distal ileum and right side of colon.
2. Ileal atresia: microcolon, non-dilated, blind-ending terminal ileal segment.
3. Meconium plug syndrome: large cast of meconium mainly in the region of the splenic flexure, small left colon.
4. Hirschsprung's disease: abrupt transition from narrow distal to dilated proximal colon. The transition is commonly at the rectosigmoid junction, but sometimes as high as the splenic flexure. Rarely, the entire colon is involved and is small.
5. Colonic atresia: blind-ending small colon.
6. Anorectal malformations: these are diagnosed clinically and can be high or low depending on whether the rectal pouch terminates above or below the level of the levator plate.

CASE 3.9: 16-YEAR-OLD BOY WITH BACK PAIN

Figure v3.9a

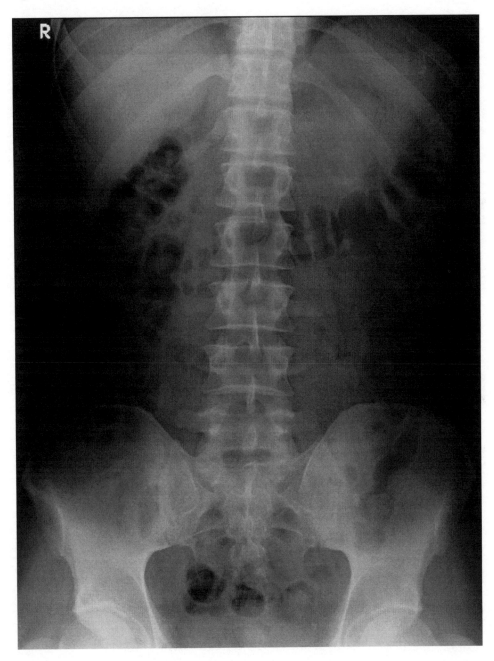

LANGERHANS CELL HISTIOCYTOSIS

FINDINGS

1. Destructive lytic lesion affecting the left twelfth rib.
2. Wide zone of transition.
3. Associated soft tissue mass.
4. No other lesions visualised.

DIFFERENTIAL DIAGNOSIS

The radiographic appearance is that of an aggressive bone lesion. In this age group, the possibilities are as follows:
1. Ewing's sarcoma
2. lymphoma
3. osteomyelitis
4. metastasis
5. Langerhans cell histiocytosis.

The patient would be unwell and pyrexial, particularly with osteomyelitis.

FURTHER INVESTIGATIONS AND MANAGEMENT

1. Review chest X-ray to look for any other rib or vertebral lesions. There may also be lung metastases, lymphoma deposits or pulmonary changes of histiocytosis.
2. CT thorax, abdomen and pelvis.
3. CT-guided biopsy of the lesion.

FURTHER INFORMATION

Lucent bone lesions are an exam favourite. The differential diagnosis is often wide. It is always best to classify them as benign or aggressive lesions. The description should include location, cortical destruction, zone of transition, soft tissue component and periosteal reaction. The fact that a lesion appears to be aggressive does not necessarily mean that it is malignant. Osteomyelitis and Langerhans cell histiocytosis are benign but can have an aggressive appearance. The above case was Langerhans cell histiocytosis.

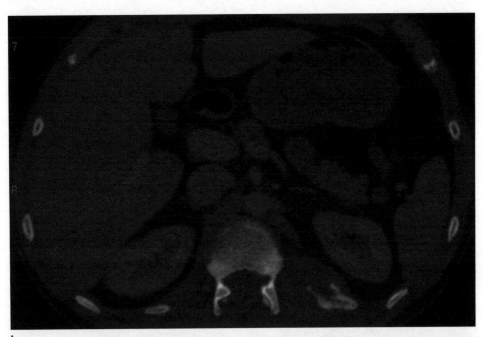

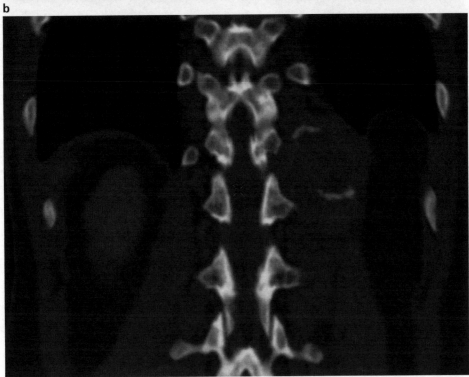

Figures v3.9b and v3.9c: Bone window axial and coronal images through the rib lesion in the above patient. There is destruction of the left twelfth rib associated with a soft tissue mass.

CASE 3.10: 45-YEAR-OLD WOMAN WITH SHORTNESS OF BREATH

Figure v3.10a

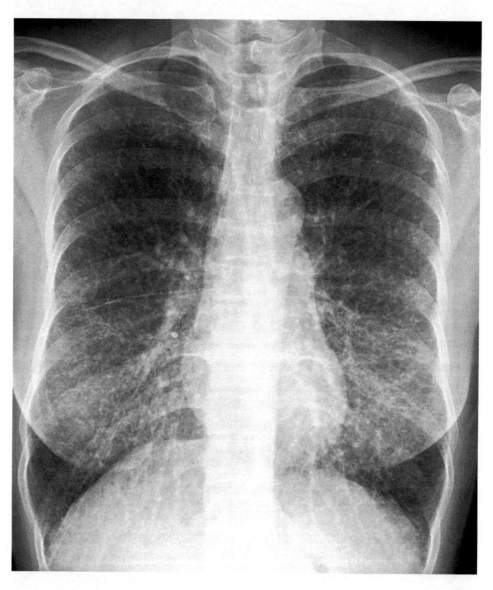

LYMPHANGIOMYOMATOSIS (LAM)

FINDINGS

1. Bilateral symmetrical diffuse coarse reticular opacification.
2. Lung volumes are increased.
3. Cardiac size and pulmonary vascularity are normal.
4. No pneumothorax or pleural effusion.

MAIN DIAGNOSIS

Lymphangiomyomatosis (LAM).

DIFFERENTIAL DIAGNOSIS

Pulmonary Langerhans cell histiocytosis (LCH). However, this is less likely as the patient is female and there is no upper to mid zone predominance of findings.

FURTHER INVESTIGATIONS AND MANAGEMENT

1. Respiratory referral.
2. HRCT of thorax.

FURTHER INFORMATION

The hallmark of LAM is cystic change of the lung parenchyma due to infiltration of the smooth muscle cells. The smooth muscle cells can also infiltrate the lymphatic system, causing lymph node enlargement and sometimes chylous pleural effusions. LAM is associated with tuberous sclerosis. Most patients present with shortness of breath, cough or pneumothorax. The condition occurs mainly in women of childbearing age, but can also occur in slightly older women. On chest X-ray, LAM appears as reticulonodular opacification with normal or increased lung volume. There may be a pneumothorax or a pleural effusion at presentation. HRCT reveals numerous thin-walled cysts of uniform size surrounded by relatively normal lung parenchyma. In contrast, the cysts are of irregular shape in LCH. Extreme lung bases tend to be spared in LCH. Nodules are more likely to occur in LCH than in LAM. LCH is associated with cigarette smoking, but no such association exists with LAM.

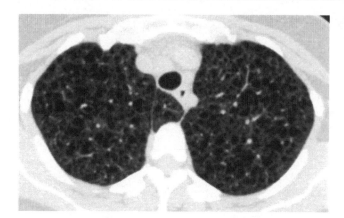

b

Figures v3.10b, v3.10c and v3.10d: HRCT in the above patient with LAM. Thin-walled uniform-sized cysts throughout both lungs. No particular basal sparing.

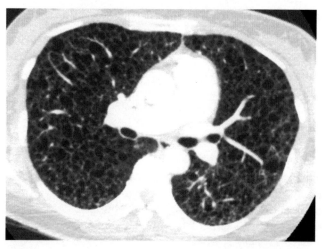

c

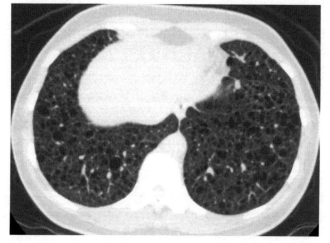

d

CASE 3.11: PREMATURE INFANT WITH ABDOMINAL DISTENSION

Figure v3.11a

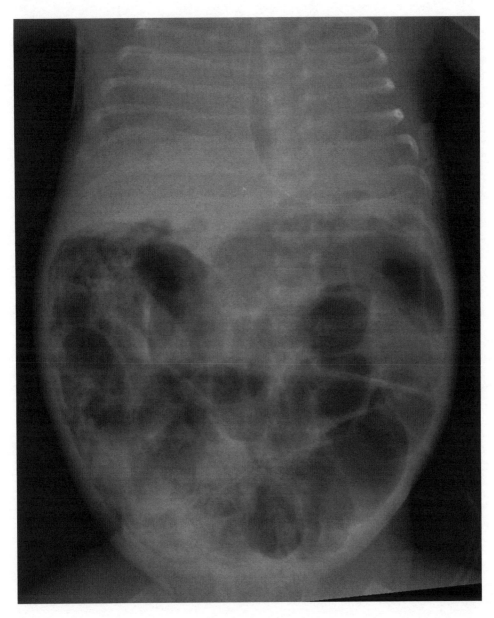

NECROTISING ENTEROCOLITIS

FINDINGS

1. The tip of the NG tube lies below the left hemidiaphragm.
2. Distended bowel loops throughout the abdomen.
3. No gas within the rectum.
4. Multiple bubbly and curvilinear lucencies seen to the right of the midline, consistent with intramural and subserosal bowel gas.
5. Portal venous gas.
6. No pneumoperitoneum.
7. Consolidation of the lower lung zones.

DIAGNOSIS

Necrotising enterocolitis with evidence of pneumatosis coli and portal venous gas.

FURTHER INVESTIGATIONS AND MANAGEMENT

Urgent surgical referral.

FURTHER INFORMATION

Necrotising enterocolitis affects primarily premature infants. Hirschsprung's disease, bowel atresias and congenital heart defects are other predispositions. Transient compromise of blood supply to the gut causes mucosal destruction, leading to submucosal gas. The terminal ileum and ascending colon are most commonly affected. Necrotising enterocolitis is treated with antibiotics and parenteral nutrition. Surgical resection may be necessary if there is bowel perforation and worsening sepsis.

CASE 3.12: 16-YEAR-OLD BOY WITH PALPABLE LUMP IN THE LEFT THIGH

Figures v3.12a, v3.12b, v3.12c, v3.12d, v3.12e, v3.12f, v3.12g and v3.12h

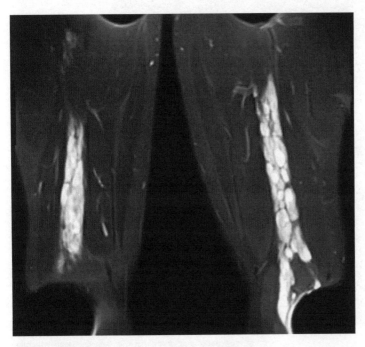

a

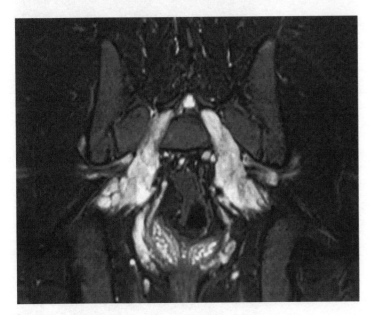

b

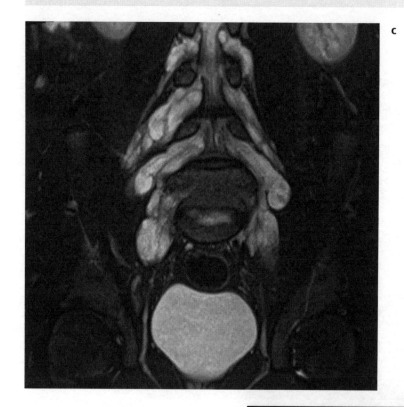

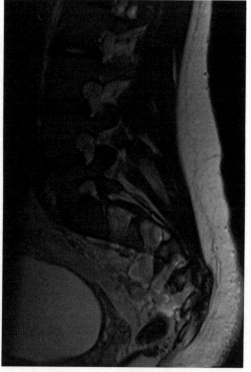

e

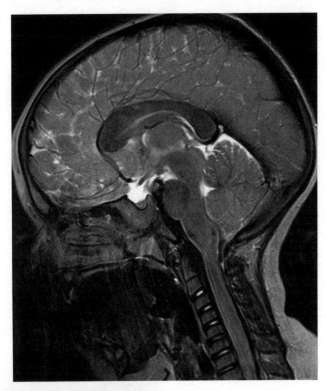

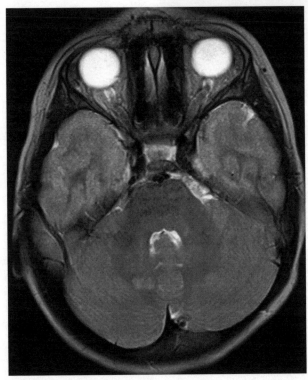

f

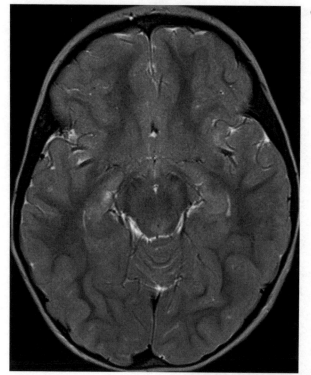

g

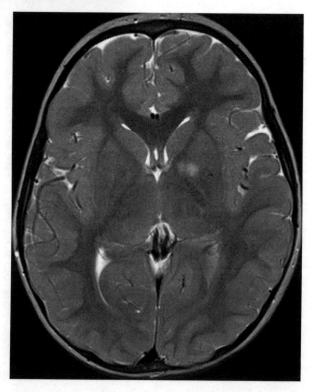

h

NEUROFIBROMATOSIS TYPE 1

FINDINGS

1. Coronal STIR images through the lumbar spine, pelvis and upper thighs and T2-weighted sagittal images through the lumbar spine:
   a. Bilateral paraspinal, lumbosacral linear high-signal masses extending into the upper thigh along the sciatic nerve distribution
   b. Widening of the neural foramina
   c. Dumb-bell-shaped masses at the sacral foramina.
2. Sagital and axial T2-weighted MRI brain:
   a. Bulky corpus callosum
   b. High-signal lesions in the dentate nuclei, right hippocampus and left lentiform nucleus with no associated mass effect
   c. Normal optic nerves.

DIAGNOSIS

Multiple plexiform neurofibromas and multiple T2-weighted high-signal areas within the brain. These findings are consistent with neurofibromatosis type 1.

FURTHER INVESTIGATIONS AND MANAGEMENT

1. Referral to neurology team.
2. Evaluation of the rest of the spine and assessment for scoliosis.

FURTHER INFORMATION

Neurofibromatosis type 1 (NF-1) is autosomal dominant with an abnormality on chromosome 17. Plexiform neurofibroma is highly suggestive of NF-1. Intracranial manifestations of NF-1 include optic pathway glioma, internal carotid artery stenosis, astrocytomas, ependymomas, meningiomas, aqueduct stenosis and heterotopias. In addition, there are often T2 bright foci within the cerebellar grey matter, basal ganglia, supratentorial white matter and brainstem which are termed neurofibromatosis bright objects (NBOs).

CASE 3.13: 33-YEAR-OLD WOMAN WITH DIPLOPIA

Figures v3.13a, v3.13b, v3.13c and v3.13d

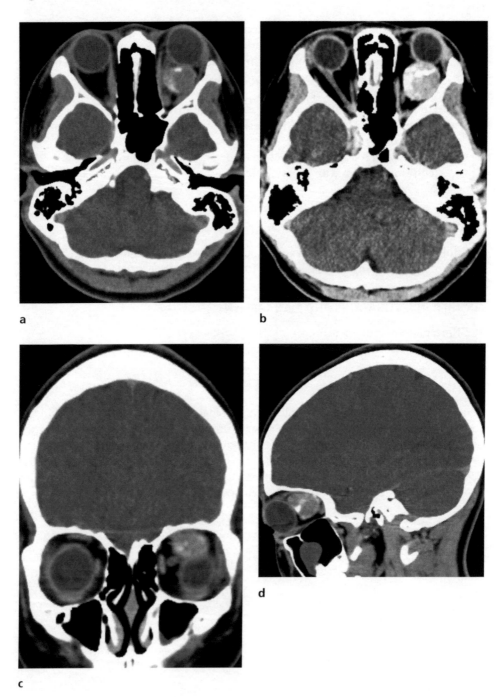

a

b

c

d

ORBITAL HAEMANGIOMA

FINDINGS

Post-contrast CT brain:
1. Well-defined, rounded enhancing left intraconal mass
2. Coarse calcifications present within the mass
3. Mass separate from the optic nerve (coronal view)
4. Mass displaces the left globe anteriorly and the extra-ocular muscles outwards
5. Extra-ocular muscles are stretched but otherwise normal
6. Orbital apex is spared.

MAIN DIAGNOSIS

Cavernous haemangioma of the left orbit.

DIFFERENTIAL DIAGNOSIS

1. Optic nerve glioma. However, this is unlikely as the mass appears to be separate from the optic nerve.
2. Inflammatory pseudotumour. However, this is unlikely as the mass is very well defined and there is no involvement of the tendons of the extra-ocular muscles or the sclera.
3. Lymphoma. However, the presence of calcifications makes this unlikely.

FURTHER INVESTIGATIONS AND MANAGEMENT

1. MRI will better delineate the relationship of the mass to the optic nerve.
2. Ophthalmology referral.

FURTHER INFORMATION

The differential diagnosis of intraconal masses is as follows:
1. orbital cavernous haemangioma
2. optic nerve glioma
3. optic nerve sheath meningioma
4. orbital pseudotumour
5. lymphoma
6. metastases
7. lymphangioma.

Orbital cavernous haemangioma is the commonest primary orbital tumour. Calcifications in cavernous haemangioma are due to phleboliths. Haemangiopericytomas are rare, but are similar in appearance to cavernous haemangiomas.

CASE 3.14: MIDDLE-AGED PATIENT WITH IRREGULAR BOWEL HABIT

Figure v3.14a

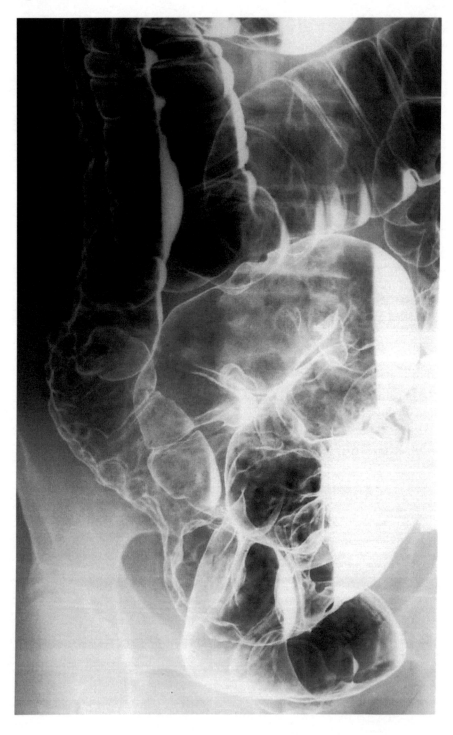

PNEUMATOSIS COLI

FINDINGS

Barium enema examination, left lateral decubitus view:
1. Multiple well-defined gas-filled cystic filling defects within the ascending colon giving rise to 'soap-bubble' appearance
2. No free gas.

MAIN DIAGNOSIS

Pneumatosis coli.

DIFFERENTIAL DIAGNOSIS

Multiple colonic polyps. However, the filling defects are lucent and of gas density – findings which indicate that these are not polyps.

FURTHER INVESTIGATIONS AND MANAGEMENT

1. Enquire whether there is a known history of cystic fibrosis, COPD or steroid intake.
2. This is a benign condition that requires no further imaging or treatment.

FURTHER INFORMATION

Causes of pneumatosis include the following:
1. Necrotising enterocolitis (in neonates): this is a serious condition that affects premature infants and can lead to bowel perforation and sepsis.
2. Steroid intake.
3. Cystic fibrosis, COPD.
4. Collagen vascular diseases.
5. Colitis: inflammatory (ulcerative colitis and Crohn's), ischaemic or infective. In this setting, gas within the bowel wall indicates bowel necrosis.

CASE 3.15: 34-YEAR-OLD MAN WITH WEIGHT LOSS AND SHORTNESS OF BREATH

Figure v3.15a

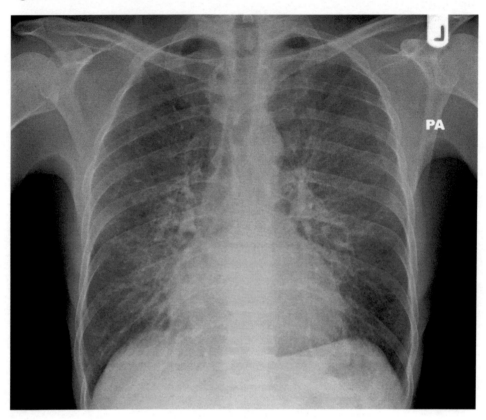

PNEUMOCYSTIS CARINII PNEUMONIA

FINDINGS

1. Bilateral, predominantly perihilar, symmetrical, ground-glass and fine interstitial opacification.
2. More focal alveolar opacification in the right lower zone.
3. Relative sparing of the bases and apices.
4. Normal heart size and pulmonary vascularity.

MAIN DIAGNOSIS

Given the history of weight loss in a young patient, pneumocystis carinii pneumonia in an immunocompromised patient is the most likely diagnosis.

DIFFERENTIAL DIAGNOSIS

Pulmonary oedema. However, this is unlikely given the absence of cardiomegaly and pleural effusions.

FURTHER INVESTIGATIONS AND MANAGEMENT

1. Sputum/bronchial lavage cytology with or without transbronchial biopsy.
2. Infectious disease referral.
3. Be alert for subsequent cystic changes and pneumothorax.

FURTHER INFORMATION

Bilateral symmetrical, perihilar or diffuse, interstitial or alveolar opacification giving rise to ground-glass change is the classical chest radiographic appearance of pneumocystis carinii pneumonia. There may be rapid development of extensive consolidation and sometimes of cysts and pneumothorax/pneumomediastinum. Pleural effusions and lymph node enlargement are uncommon findings in pneumocystis pneumonia.

CASE 3.16: 32-YEAR-OLD MAN WITH SHORTNESS OF BREATH

Figure v3.16a

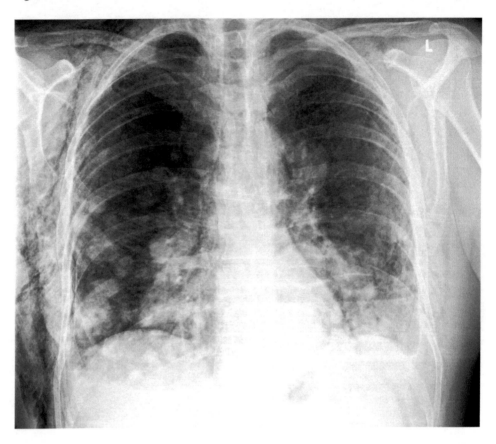

SARCOMA METASTASES: BILATERAL PNEUMOTHORACES

FINDINGS

1. Moderate-sized left hydropneumothorax.
2. Small right pneumothorax.
3. Marked surgical emphysema that is significantly worse on the right side.
4. No features to suggest tension pneumothorax.
5. Multiple bilateral soft tissue density pulmonary nodules including large left hilar and retrocardiac lung masses.
6. Visible bones unremarkable.

DIAGNOSIS

Multiple bilateral pulmonary metastases, left hydropneumothorax, right pneumothorax and extensive surgical emphysema. In view of the spontaneous pneumothoraces, the metastases are likely to be secondary to a sarcoma.

FURTHER INVESTIGATIONS AND MANAGEMENT

1. Medical referral for urgent chest drain insertion.
2. CT chest, abdomen and pelvis and thorough search for primary sarcoma.

FURTHER INFORMATION

Metastatic sarcomas can cavitate secondary to necrosis, resulting in pneumothorax. Pneumothorax occurs with sarcomas and other aggressive necrotic tumours. It occurs most frequently with osteosarcoma. Necrosis of peripheral subpleural metastases is thought to be the cause of such pneumothoraces. A spontaneous pneumothorax in a patient with a known sarcoma raises the possibility of pulmonary metastases.

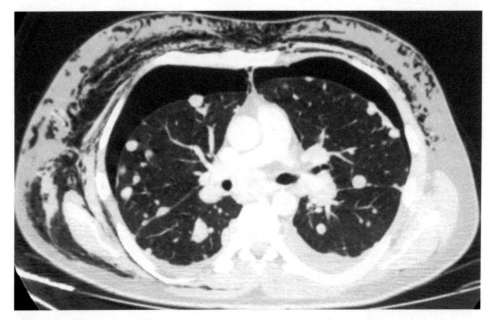

Figure v3.16b: CT scan of thorax in the above patient confirming bilateral pneumothoraces, multiple lung metastases and marked surgical emphysema. Also note the small bilateral pleural effusions.

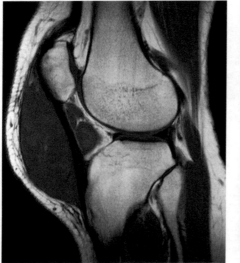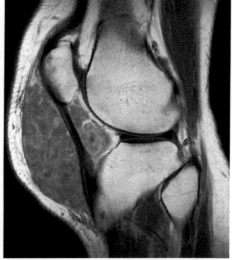

Figures v3.16c and v3.16d: T1 pre- and post-contrast sagittal knee MRI showing a large enhancing infrapatellar soft tissue mass extending into the Hoffa's fat pad. Diagnosis was soft tissue sarcoma.

CASE 3.17: 55-YEAR-OLD MAN WITH A HISTORY OF DIARRHOEA AND RECTAL BLEEDING

Figures v3.17a and v3.17b

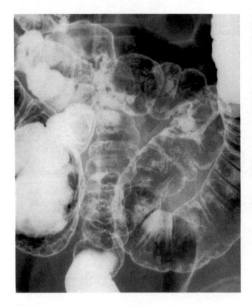

a

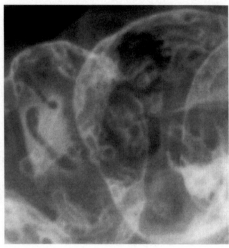

b

POST-INFLAMMATORY PSEUDOPOLYPS

FINDINGS

Double-contrast barium enema study:
1. Well-defined filiform linear and bridging filling defects throughout the colon
2. Normal haustral pattern.

MAIN DIAGNOSIS

Post-inflammatory polyposis, most probably secondary to previous ulcerative colitis.

DIFFERENTIAL DIAGNOSIS

Post-inflammatory polyposis due to Crohn's disease.

FURTHER INVESTIGATIONS AND MANAGEMENT

If there is any clinical concern, colonoscopy and biopsy must be performed to exclude the possibility of a malignant lesion.

FURTHER INFORMATION

In long-standing pancolitis, the bowel wall can shorten. This leads to the formation of pseudopolyps, which are areas of normal or hypertrophied mucosa within areas of atrophy. Post-inflammatory pseudopolyps are not dysplastic polyps and are therefore not a risk factor for colonic cancer. However, they may complicate recognition of true adenomas and dysplasia-associated lesion or mass (DALM). If there is any clinical concern, colonoscopy and biopsy should be recommended.

CASE 3.18: NEONATE WITH LEG SIZE DISCREPANCY

Figure v3.18a

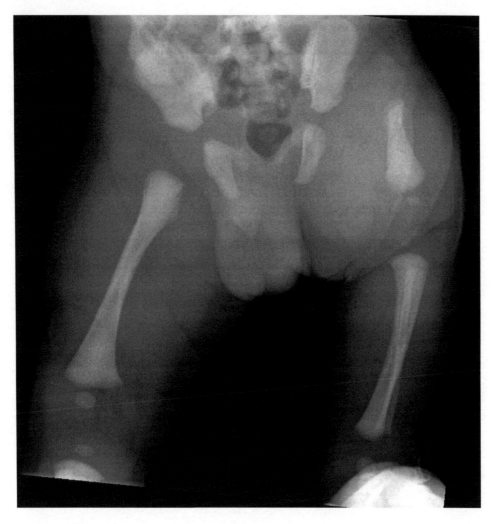

PROXIMAL FEMORAL FOCAL DEFICIENCY

FINDINGS

1. The left femur is shortened and deformed.
2. The left femoral head is dislocated superolaterally.
3. Hypoplastic left lower femoral and upper tibial epiphyses compared with the right.
4. The left tibia and fibula are of normal length.

DIAGNOSIS

Proximal femoral focal deficiency.

FURTHER INVESTIGATIONS AND MANAGEMENT

Orthopaedic referral.

FURTHER INFORMATION

Proximal femoral focal deficiency (PFFD) is secondary to failure of normal development of the proximal femur. A short femur is present which is laterally and superiorly displaced. A variable length of the proximal femur is hypoplastic, but the distal femur is more or less present. In severe form, the femur may be completely absent. Other associated features that may be present are coxa vara, hypoplastic knee, hypoplastic fibula, ankle deformities and absent rays.

CASE 3.19: ABDOMINAL DISTENSION

Figure v3.19a

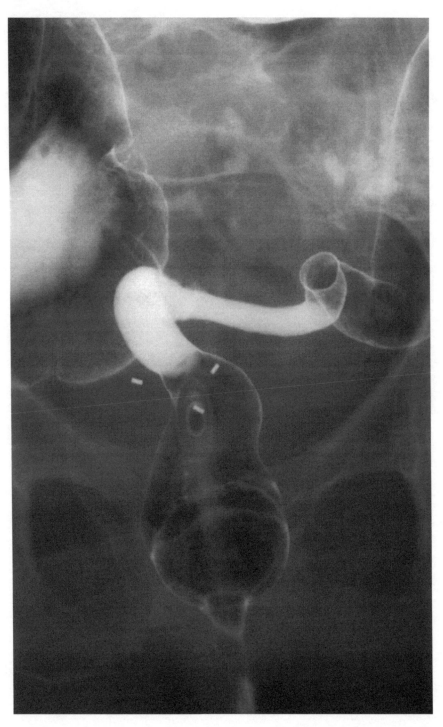

RADIATION STRICTURE

FINDINGS

Double-contrast barium enema examination, frontal sigmoid view:
1. Smooth narrowing of a long segment of sigmoid colon
2. Three metallic radiotherapy markers within the pelvis.

MAIN DIAGNOSIS

Smooth sigmoid colonic stricture secondary to previous radiotherapy.

DIFFERENTIAL DIAGNOSIS

Ischaemic stricture. However, this is less likely as ischaemic strictures tend to be irregular, with associated large sacculations.

FURTHER INVESTIGATIONS AND MANAGEMENT

1. Establish the history of previous pelvic radiotherapy.
2. Sigmoidoscopy and biopsy.

FURTHER INFORMATION

Rectosigmoid stricture is a late complication of pelvic irradiation for cancers of the cervix, prostate, testes and bladder. The median interval for development of radiation colitis is 2 years. Colitis is secondary to ischaemia as a result of obliterative endarteritis which is followed by fibrosis. The strictures appear as generalised narrowing within the radiation field. Metallic radiotherapy markers are a clue to the diagnosis.

CASE 3.20: 10-YEAR-OLD GIRL WITH SEIZURES

Figures v3.20a, v3.20b, v3.20c and v3.20d

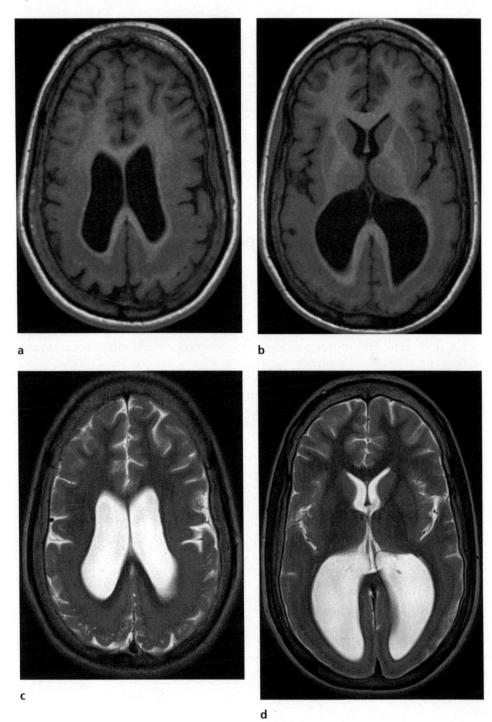

a

b

c

d

SUBCORTICAL BAND HETEROTOPIA

FINDINGS

MRI brain, T1- and T2-weighted axial images:
1. Abnormal gyral pattern and symmetrical loss of cortical sulcation along the temporal, parietal and occipital lobes
2. Thinning of the parieto-occipital cortex
3. Bilateral thick band of heterotopic grey matter located between the ventricular walls and cortex, with interpositioned thin bands of white matter
4. Colpocephaly
5. Normal frontal lobes, basal ganglia and corpus callosum.

DIAGNOSIS

Subcortical band heterotopia.

FURTHER INVESTIGATIONS AND MANAGEMENT

Neurology referral.

FURTHER INFORMATION

Heterotopias are abnormalities of neuronal migration from germinal matrix to the cerebral cortex. Heterotopic grey matter is located in the wrong place, and there are consequent seizures and developmental delay.

There are two main types of heterotopias, namely nodular and band. Nodular heterotopias can be either subependymal or subcortical. There is a female preponderance of heterotopias. Heterotopias can be associated with complete or partial agenesis of the corpus callosum.

CASE 3.21: 56-YEAR-OLD WITH WEIGHT LOSS

Figure v3.21a

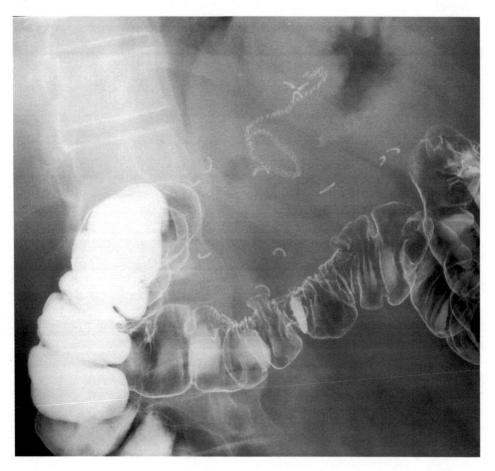

SUBMUCOSAL METASTASES FROM GASTRIC CANCER

FINDINGS

Double-contrast barium enema study, showing the transverse colon:
1. Multiple surgical clips projected within the upper abdomen
2. Surgical suture line in the left upper quadrant suggestive of previous gastric surgery and anastomosis
3. Mild narrowing of a long segment of transverse colon with irregular crenellated superior mucosal surface.

MAIN DIAGNOSIS

Colonic spread of gastric cancer through the gastrocolic ligament.

DIFFERENTIAL DIAGNOSIS

Primary colonic carcinoma with a history of previous gastric surgery.

FURTHER INVESTIGATIONS AND MANAGEMENT

1. CT chest, abdomen and pelvis for staging.
2. Upper GI endoscopy with or without colonoscopy and biopsy.

FURTHER INFORMATION

Gastric carcinoma can invade the transverse colon via the gastrocolic ligament, and pancreatic carcinoma can invade it via the transverse mesocolon. The former causes irregularity and a crenellated appearance at the superior border and the latter causes this appearance at the inferior border of the transverse colon.

Further reading

JOURNALS

Berrocal T, Madrid C, Nova S *et al.* Congenital anomalies of the tracheobronchial tree, lung and mediastinum: embryology, radiology and pathology. *Radiographics.* 2004; **24:** e17.

Flach HZ, Ginai AZ, Oosterhuis JW. Maffucci syndrome: radiologic and pathologic findings. *Radiographics.* 2001; **21:** 1311–16.

Furrer M, Althaus U, Ris HB. Spontaneous pneumothorax from radiographically occult metastatic sarcoma. *Eur J Cardiothorac Surg.* 1997; **11:** 1171–3.

Goldstraw P. The 7th edition of TNM in lung cancer: what now? *J Thorac Oncol.* 2009; **4:** 671–3.

Horton KM, Lawler LP, Fishman EK. CT findings in sclerosing mesenteritis (panniculitis): spectrum of disease. *Radiographics.* 2003; **23:** 1561–7.

Husain AN, Hessel RG. Neonatal pulmonary hypoplasia: an autopsy study of 25 cases. *Pediatr Pathol.* 1993; **13:** 475–84.

Iafrate F, Laghi A, Paolantonio P *et al.* Preoperative staging of rectal cancer with MR imaging: correlation with surgical and histopathological findings. *Radiographics.* 2006; **26:** 701–14.

Libshitz HI, North LB. Pulmonary metastases. *Radiol Clin North Am.* 1982; **20:** 437–51.

Seo JB, Im JG, Goo JM *et al.* Atypical pulmonary metastases: spectrum of radiological findings. *Radiographics.* 2001; **21:** 403–17.

White JS, Skelly RT, Gardiner KR *et al.* Intravasation of barium sulphate at barium enema examination. *Br J Radiol.* 2006; **79:** e32–5.

BOOKS

Adam A, Dixon AK. *Grainger and Allison's Diagnostic Radiology: a textbook of medical imaging.* 5th edn. Churchill Livingstone; 2008.

Braunwald E, Fauci A, Kasper DL *et al. Harrison's Principles of Internal Medicine.* 15th edn. McGraw-Hill; 2001.

Chapman S, Nakielny R. *Aids to Radiological Differential Diagnosis.* 4th edn. Saunders; 2003.

Dahnert W. *Radiological Review Manual.* 5th edn. Lippincott Williams & Wilkins; 2003.

de Lacey G, Morley S, Berman L. *The Chest X-ray Survival Guide.* Saunders Elsevier; 2008.

Gay S, Woodcock RJ. *Radiology Recall.* Lippincott Williams & Wilkins; 2000.

Grossman RI, Yousem DM. *Neuroradiology: the requisites.* 2nd edn. Mosby; 2003.

Harnsberger HR. *Handbook of Head and Neck Imaging.* 2nd edn. Mosby; 1995.

Haslett C, Chilvers ER, Boon NA *et al. Davidson's Principles and Practice of Medicine*. 19th edn. Churchill Livingstone; 2002.

Helms CA. *Fundamentals of Skeletal Radiology*. 3rd edn. Elsevier; 2005.

Helms CA, Major NM, Anderson MW *et al. Musculoskeletal MRI*. 2nd edn. Saunders; 2009.

Lee JKT, Sagel SS, Stanley RJ *et al. Computed Body Tomography with MRI Correlation*. 4th edn. Lippincott Williams & Wilkins; 2006.

Pitman AG, Major NM, Tello R. *Radiology Core Review*. Saunders; 2003.

Seaton A, Seaton D. *Crofton and Douglas's Respiratory Diseases*. 5th edn. Blackwell Science; 2000.

Semelka RC. *Abdominal–Pelvic MRI*. 2nd edn. Wiley-Liss; 2006.

Staatz G, Honnef D, Piroth W *et al. Direct Diagnosis in Radiology Paediatric Imaging*. Thieme; 2008.

Sutton D. *Textbook of Radiology and Imaging*. 7th edn. Churchill Livingstone; 2003.

Webb WR, Muller NL, Naidich DP. *High-Resolution CT of the Lung*. 4th edn. Lippincott Williams & Wilkins; 2009.

Weissleder R, Wittenberg J, Harisinghani M. *Primer of Diagnostic Imaging*. 3rd edn. Mosby; 2003.

WEBSITE

Royal College of Radiologists. *Final FRCR Part B Examination*. www.rcr.ac.uk/content.aspx?PageID=725 (accessed 16 August 2010).

Index